Copyright © 2012-2022 FlightBridgeED, LLC. All rights reserved.

No part of this book may be reproduced in any form, printed or electronic, without written permission of the copyright holder.

The views expressed herein are those of the authors and do not necessarily reflect the views of your employer, medical director or current protocols.

This publication is intended to provide accurate information regarding the subject matter addressed herein. However, it is published with the understanding that FlightBridgeED, LLC is not authorizing or advising you to engage in unsafe practice or render care above your current state or county protocols. The information contained herein is solely for advanced education for licensed professionals wishing to further their knowledge base. It is not intended for the layperson to provide medical care. It should not supersede each individual's scope of practice or current medical policies and procedures for which the individual is covered under. It is the individuals' responsibility to use their own clinical judgment for decision-making and provide care in a manner consistent with current standards of care. The information in this publication is subject to change at any time without notice based on new research or treatment approaches that are standard in the medical industry. Neither FlightBridgeED, LLC nor the authors of the publication, make any guarantees or warranties concerning the information contained herein. Readers are urged to review current package indications and usage guidelines and protocols provided by the manufacturers of the agents mentioned.

First Edition Printing – October 2017
Updated July 2022
FlightBridgeED, LLC
Headquarters
Bowling Green, KY
Phone + 1 800-991-3160
www.flightbridgeed.com

platelet admin → 1u/10kg body weight
b) dont give in ITP/TTP/DIC

FlightBridgeED, LLC

Subfalcine herniation ≅ midline shift

Table of Contents

Preface 2

Chapter 1 - Oxygenation, Acids & Alkalis 3

Chapter 2 - Respiratory – Breathing & Wheezing 10

Chapter 3 - Ventilation, Ventilators & "Baby Lungs" 14

Chapter 4 - Flight Physiology 21

Chapter 5 - Little Tikes, Heat & Cold Injuries 24

Chapter 6 - Hematology & Electrolytes 28

Chapter 7 - Little Hearts - RPMs & PUMP 32

Chapter 8 - Endocrine & Renal – Hormones & Pee 39

Chapter 9 - Trauma – Trips, Spills, Breaks & Catastrophes .. 44

Chapter 10 - Neurological Emergencies 51

Chapter 11 - Toxicology – Poisons & Toxic Ingestions 54

Chapter 12 - Neonatal Defects - Surgical Emergencies 58

Chapter 13 - Lab Values Dissected 65

Chapter 14 - Review Question Rationale 74

Chapter 15 - Study Tips 124

References.. 125

Cyanotic → need ductal flow
  → low SaO₂, worsens w/ O₂, need PGE1
acyanotic → vent inflow or outflow obstruction
  → causes fluid back-up ∘ CHF

Handwritten notes at top:

Δ 10mmHg PaCO₂ — pH 0.08 ↓↑
Δ 10 mEq/L HCO₃⁻ — pH 0.15 ↓↓ ↑↑
Δ pH 0.10 — K⁺ 0.6 ↓↑

Preface

FlightBridgeED, LLC is a "live" and online educational organization that specializes in providing critical care transition education for the individual wanting to move from ground E.M.S., the Emergency Department, or Intensive Care Unit to the helicopter E.M.S. (HEMS) industry. The project was founded in November 2012 as the product of the combined visions of the FlightBridgeED team. The idea for FlightBridgeED started as a casual conversation and a subsequent formal meeting which resulted in several podcast recordings and an initial deployment of the website. As a community began to develop around the project, the team saw opportunities for improvement and expansion in order to better serve those interested in this very specialized type of education. Listening to YOUR feedback, FlightBridgeED has expanded its vision to develop a complete, multifaceted **"Live" & Online Education System** designed to bridge the gap between ground based healthcare and the air medical industry; A Partnership in Discovery™.

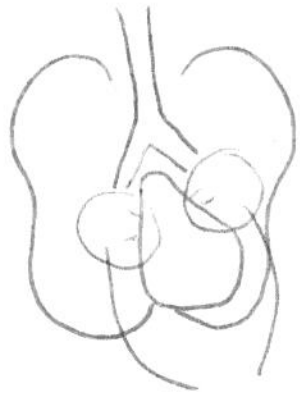

Handwritten margin notes: hilar area (hilum) → pulm art & veins coming off

Throughout the past 16 years working in the HEMS industry, there have been many strides made industry wide to bring good quality critical care education to the thousands of Flight Nurses and Paramedics worldwide. Since the inception of FlightBridgeED, we have been driven to bring the best education materials to the industry that meets and exceeds the national standards in critical care.

The goal of this book is to provide the most up to date information based on experience, knowledge and current research studies that will make you prepared to take these challenging exams. Whether you are preparing to take the C-NPT, CFRN, FP-C, CCP-C or CTRN, we at FlightBridgeED feel like our educational materials will greatly assist you in becoming credentialed in your specific discipline. We feel this separates us from other companies and will make you, the "student", more successful in your testing and career goals. We not only want you to pass these exams, but also want to make you better clinicians and health care providers.

Handwritten notes at bottom:

GOLDMARK → metabolic acidosis causes

metabolic acidosis without anion gap means the cause is loss of bicarb

milrinone > dobutamine if pt has pulm HTN

vaso bolus → 1-2 units q 2-3 min
prostaglandin admin → risk for apnea

FlightBridgeED, LLC

Chapter 1 | Oxygenation, Acids & Alkalis

1) Your 3-year-old pediatric patient's current ABGs are:

pH 7.30, $PaCO_2$ 24, PaO_2 62, HCO_3^- 16. What is your interpretation?

a. Uncompensated respiratory acidosis
b. Uncompensated metabolic acidosis
c. Partially compensated metabolic acidosis
d. Partially compensated respiratory acidosis

2) Your 6-year-old pediatric patient's current ABGs are:

pH 7.55, $PaCO_2$ 30, PaO_2 56, HCO_3^- 25. What is your interpretation?

a. Uncompensated respiratory alkalosis
b. Uncompensated respiratory acidosis
c. Compensated respiratory acidosis
d. Compensated respiratory alkalosis

3) Your 12-year-old pediatric patient has a pH of 7.52. Their previous pH was 7.41 and their potassium (K^+) was 4.7mEq/L. You would expect the current K+ to be approximately?

a. 5.3 mEq/L
b. 5.5 mEq/L
c. 3.9 mEq/L
d. 4.1 mEq/L

4) Your 8-year-old pediatric patient's initial ABG values are: pH 7.25, $PaCO_2$ 51, PaO_2 104, HCO_3^- 27, SpO_2 97%, $EtCO_2$ 54. You have had the patient on your transport ventilator during your one-hour flight. Now their $EtCO_2$ is showing 34. You would anticipate which of the following?

a. pH 7.43
b. pH 7.42
c. pH 7.41
d. pH 7.40

5) The Bohr effect states?

   a. In the presence of decreased pH or increased acid, the hemoglobin (Hgb) will release its load of O_2 to the tissues
   b. States of high oxygen concentrations enhances the unloading of carbon dioxide
   c. The lungs can adjust the amount of carbonic acid by blowing off or holding onto carbon dioxide
   d. Lactate levels are directly proportional to mortality and for every point above 2.5, mortality increases by 10%

6) Your patient's current lactate level is 6.3mmol/L. This value suggests?

   a. A state of metabolic acidosis is present and a state of shock is imminent
   b. Nothing, as this test has been proven to be non-beneficial
   c. Aerobic metabolism is occurring and a desirable state for homeostasis is present
   d. Stress response indicator and can be used as a biomarker for morbidity and mortality

7) When using the "Winters formula" to calculate the effects of $PaCO_2$ on pH, you know that for every 10mmHg change in CO_2, the pH will change by _____ in the opposite direction?

   a. 0.09
   b. 0.06
   c. 0.08
   d. 0.10

8) You are transporting a 6-year-old with current ABGs of: pH 7.37, $PaCO_2$ 58, $HCO3^-$ 23, Base deficit -2, PaO_2 106. What is your current diagnosis?

   a. Compensated metabolic acidosis
   b. Compensated respiratory acidosis
   c. Compensated respiratory alkalosis
   d. Compensated metabolic alkalosis

FlightBridgeED, LLC

9) You are flying a 3-year-old pediatric patient in respiratory distress secondary to respiratory syncytial virus (RSV). You know the earliest stages of shock most likely will present with which acid-base disorder?

    a. Metabolic acidosis
    b. Respiratory acidosis
    c. Respiratory alkalosis
    d. Metabolic alkalosis

10) When applying rules from the "Winters formula", you know that a change in HCO_3^- of 10 mEq, will change the pH _____ in the same direction?

    a. 0.10
    b. 0.15
    c. 0.08
    d. 0.06

11) Identify your 1-year-old pediatric patient's following ABGs: pH 7.6, $PaCO_2$ 23, HCO_3^- 35, PaO_2 85.

    a. Respiratory acidosis
    b. Respiratory alkalosis
    c. Metabolic alkalosis
    d. Mixed disturbance

12) You have the following ABG readings: pH 7.10, $PaCO_2$ 50 mmHg, HCO_3^- 24, PaO_2 92, $EtCO_2$ 50 mmHg, SpO_2 92%. You are attempting to manipulate the pH by increasing the patient's minute ventilation (V_E) on the transport ventilator. If you increase the V_E to reflect a decrease in $EtCO_2$ from 50 mmHg down to 30 mmHg, what would your change in pH reflect?

    a. pH 7.08
    b. pH 7.26
    c. pH 7.12
    d. pH 7.30

13) You are enroute to receive a multi-systems trauma patient. You receive their current ABG results. Which of the following blood gas results would have you preparing to intubate and ventilate the patient?

    a. pH 7.38, $PaCO_2$ 44, PaO_2 84, HCO_3^- 20
    b. pH 7.35, $PaCO_2$ 48, PaO_2 80, HCO_3^- 26
    c. pH 7.03, $PaCO_2$ 75, PaO_2 50, HCO_3^- 16
    d. pH 7.05, $PaCO_2$ 15, PaO_2 158, HCO_3^- 8

14) In metabolic acidosis, which electrolyte becomes falsely elevated due to the acid-base disorder?

   a. Calcium
   b. Chloride
   c. Potassium
   d. Sodium

15) Your 8-year-old pediatric patient has traumatic injuries secondary to abuse. The patient has received 3 units of PRBCs. You would anticipate the patient's 2,3-DPG to change and cause the oxyhemoglobin dissociation curve to shift to?

   a. Stay the same as 2,3-DPG has no effect on the oxyhemoglobin dissociation curve
   b. Shift to the right
   c. Shift upward, thus increasing the patient's oxygenation status
   d. Shift to the left

16) You are transporting a 9-year-old pediatric patient from a local ICU. You note the patient has consistent NG suctioning and confirm this with the patient's referring RN. Based on this, you would expect what acid-base disorder?

   a. Respiratory acidosis
   b. Respiratory alkalosis
   c. Metabolic acidosis
   d. Metabolic alkalosis

17) A 3-year-old, 20kg, patient who had a recent traumatic injury secondary to an MVC and is suffering from aspiration pneumonia. They are unresponsive and intubated and have the following vitals: BP 78/40, HR 110, RR 20/assisted. They are mechanically ventilated and have no spontaneous respirations. Dopamine is infusing at 10mcg/kg/min. Current ventilator settings are: SIMV 20 PC 10, V$_{te}$ 112, f 26, PEEP 5 and FiO$_2$ 0.6. Current ABGs: pH 7.34, PaCO$_2$ 50 mmHg, HCO3$^-$ 19, PaO$_2$ 50, and SpO$_2$ 90%. What would your next treatment priority be?

   a. Increase the FiO$_2$ and PEEP to 8 cmH$_2$0
   b. Wean the Dopamine to 7.5 mcg/kg/min
   c. Continue transporting with no additional interventions
   d. Provide a fluid bolus of 250mL LR

18) Oxygen saturation (SpO_2) refers to the % of oxygen that is?

   a. Carried by both plasma and Hgb
   b. Bound to Hgb
   c. Dissolved in the plasma
   d. Also known as oxygen carrying capacity

19) Identify the following ABG:

   pH 7.28, $PaCO_2$ 20, $HCO3^-$ 17, PaO_2 80, BE -8

   a. Mixed disturbance
   b. Compensated metabolic acidosis
   c. Partially compensated metabolic acidosis
   d. Uncompensated metabolic acidosis

20) Acute respiratory failure is defined as?

   a. PaO_2 < 80 and a $PaCO_2$ > 45
   b. PaO_2 < 70 and a $PaCO_2$ > 60
   c. PaO_2 < 60 and a $PaCO_2$ > 50
   d. PaO_2 < 50 and a $PaCO_2$ > 45

21) A shift to the right on the oxyhemoglobin dissociation curve can be caused by?

   a. Alkalosis
   b. Hypothermia
   c. Decreased levels of 2,3-DPG
   d. Hyperthermia

22) Which condition would result in a left shift on the oxyhemoglobin dissociation curve?

   a. pH of 7.10
   b. $PaCO_2$ of 55 mmHg
   c. Decreased levels of 2,3-DPG
   d. A temperature of 103.0 F

23) Why would a patient experience cellular hypoxia during massive transfusions of PRBCs?

   a. Metabolic acidosis
   b. Hemolytic reaction
   c. Decreased levels of 2,3-DPG
   d. Decreased calcium levels

24) All of the following cause altered states of the oxyhemoglobin dissociation curve EXCEPT?

a. pH
b. 2,3-DPG Levels
c. Massive transfusions with PRBCs
d. Decreased cardiac output

25) Identify the following formula:

$$CO_2 + H_2O \leftrightarrow H_2CO_3 \leftrightarrow HCO_3^- + H^+$$

a. Acid-base balance
b. Bicarbonate buffer system
c. Regulation of H^+
d. Glycolysis

26) Causes of metabolic alkalosis include all of the following EXCEPT?

a. Decreased levels of potassium (K^+)
b. Decreased levels of chloride (Cl^-)
c. Retention of hydrogen (H^+)
d. Increased magnesium (Mg^{++})

27) Your patient is demonstrating an increase in venous oxygen saturation (SvO_2) and decrease in oxygen consumption (VO_2) and pH. What type of shock do you suspect?

a. Anaphylactic
b. Cardiogenic
c. Hemorrhagic
d. Septic

28) This equation is used to identify what?

$$[1.34 \times Hgb \times (SaO_2)] + PaO_2 \times 0.003$$

a. Oxygen content in the arteries
b. Oxygen uptake by the cells
c. Amount of oxygen bound to Hgb
d. Oxygen uptake by the muscle

29) Your patient is a 1-year-old with left upper lobe pneumonia. Current vitals: BP 70/36, HR 138, RR 48, SpO$_2$ 87% and T 102.1°F. Current ABG: pH 7.20, PaCO$_2$ 68, HCO3$^-$ 32, PaO$_2$ 50. This presentation will result in which of the following changes?

       a. Right shift with decreased SaO$_2$
       b. Left shift with increased SaO$_2$
       c. Right shift with increased SaO$_2$
       d. Left shift with decreased SaO$_2$

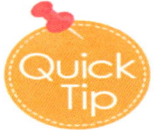

Bohr effect – In the presence of increased acid, the Hgb will lose its affinity for oxygen and will dump it to the tissues. This will cause a high PaO$_2$ and lower SaO$_2$!

Chapter 2 | Respiratory – Breathing & Wheezing

1) Which of the following does not have bronchodilation effects?

   a. Albuterol
   b. Terbutaline
   c. Decadron
   d. Ketamine

2) A 3-hour-old neonate is found to be polycythemic. What is the likely cause?

   a. Normal HbF
   b. Placental transfusion
   c. Fetal anemia
   d. Low amniotic fluid level

3) You perform a needle thoracostomy on your neonate with a suspected "air leak". After re-evaluating the neonate, which of the following would indicate that your treatment was NOT successful?

   a. An increase in the MAP from 54 to 76 after the procedure
   b. A sudden rush of air coming from the needle after the procedure
   c. A decrease in the respiratory rate from 36 to 24 after the procedure
   d. A shift of the trachea away from the needle after the procedure

4) You are administering Albuterol to a 4-year-old. Which of the following changes would NOT be anticipated with administration?

   a. Bronchodilation
   b. Tachycardia
   c. Tingling in extremities
   d. Hypertension

5) You are preparing your 30-week gestation, 1.5kg, neonate for transfer. The patient was delivered 3 hours ago. The referring RN shows you the patient's current chest x-ray. You note a ground glass appearance on the chest film. Your current vent settings are: SIMV 26, PRVC, Vte 8, f 48 FiO_2 0.21 and PEEP 5. Current ABG: pH 7.24, $PaCO_2$ 38, PaO_2 40, HCO_3^- 24. What condition do you suspect?

   a. Hyaline membrane disease
   b. Tetralogy of Fallot
   c. Cor pulmonale
   d. Pulmonary edema

FlightBridgeED, LLC

6) A 6-year-old is complaining of increasing dyspnea, non-productive cough and fever. The mother states the patient had a loud "barking cough". Current vitals: BP 78/38, HR 146, RR 36, SpO_2 92% on room air. Based upon your assessment, what would your initial diagnosis be for this patient?

    a. Pneumocystis pneumonia (PCP)
    b. Spontaneous pneumothorax
    c. Respiratory syncytial virus (RSV)
    d. Croup

7) Which medication is recommended for sedation in a patient with asthma?

    a. Etomidate
    b. Fentanyl
    c. Versed
    d. Ketamine

8) What is your priority when treating respiratory acidosis?

    a. Improve oxygenation by placing the patient on a non-rebreather (NRB)
    b. Administer sodium bicarbonate to buffer the acid
    c. Improve alveolar ventilation by reversing the cause of hypoventilation
    d. Administer an anxiolytic to decrease anxiety and improve oxygenation

9) Which of the following can be associated with a poor prognosis in a patient with severe acute respiratory syndrome (ARDS)?

    a. Fever >103.0°F
    b. Leukocytosis
    c. Elevated lactate
    d. Increased CO_2

10) Oxygen delivery (DO_2) is a product of what?

    a. PaO_2, MAP, SvO_2
    b. SaO_2, Hgb, CO
    c. PaO_2, Hgb, MAP
    d. SvO_2, CI, SaO_2

11) You are called to transport a 4-year-old who is in respiratory distress. They are anxious appearing and you are told that they have a past medical history of asthma. Current vitals are: BP 80/32, HR 130, RR 38. You auscultate crackles throughout. You place the patient on your monitor and note sinus tachycardia. You ask if ABGs have currently been obtained and the transferring RN goes to check. You would anticipate which of the following findings on the ABGs?

    a. Decreased pH, increased $PaCO_2$, normal PaO_2
    b. Decreased pH, increased $PaCO_2$, decreased PaO_2
    c. Increased pH, decreased $PaCO_2$, decreased PaO_2
    d. Increased pH, decreased $PaCO_2$, normal PaO_2

12) You have responded to a fire in a building with two pediatric victims. The patients are exhibiting worsening respiratory distress and cough after high flow O_2 had been applied. What may be causing the patient's signs/symptoms?

    a. Cyanide
    b. Ammonia
    c. Carbon dioxide
    d. Hydrocarbon

13) You are in-flight with a 30-week gestation neonate with a hypoplastic left heart. The neonate is on FiO_2 of 18% with a corresponding pre-ductal SpO_2 of 71%. You are at 2,000 feet and the patient has an increase in SpO_2 to 73%. What is your initial intervention for this patient?

    a. Decrease oxygen delivery to the patient
    b. Increase oxygen delivery to the patient
    c. RSI and intubate the patient
    d. Identify and correct the FiO_2 based on the new barometric pressure

14) When evaluating a patient in acute respiratory failure, identify the most common finding?

    a. Epistaxis
    b. $PaO_2 > 100$ mmHg
    c. $PaCO_2 > 50$ mmHg
    d. Pulmonary fibrosis

15) When pre-oxygenating your 4-year-old rapid sequence intubation (RSI) patient, you know the strategy for doing so is?

    a. Displacing the CO_2
    b. Causing nitrogen washout
    c. Increasing alveolar shunting
    d. Decreasing alveolar shunting

16) The proper depth of a 3.5 endotracheal tube (ETT) would be?

    a. 10.5 cm
    b. 11 cm
    c. 12 cm
    d. 14 cm

17) You are transporting a 48-week post conceptual age infant. The baby is being transported for RSV. You know this puts the infant at higher risk for?

    a. Bradycardia
    b. Tachycardia
    c. Tachypnea
    d. Apnea

18) In regards to the above infant with respiratory syncytial virus (RSV), the best treatment combination is?

    a. Nebulized Atrovent and suctioning
    b. Nebulized normal saline and suctioning
    c. Nebulized Albuterol and suctioning
    d. Nebulized Atropine and suctioning

Chapter 3 | Ventilation, Ventilators & "Baby Lungs"

1) Your patient is demonstrating a sudden elevated PIP with a normal Pplat. The most likely cause is?

   a. Asthma
   b. ARDS
   c. Pulmonary edema
   d. Tension pneumothorax

2) The main disadvantage of pressure-limited ventilation is?

   a. High FiO_2 is required for adequate oxygenation
   b. PEEP cannot be used due to the potential for barotrauma
   c. You do not have a guaranteed minute ventilation (V_E) and higher risk for hypoventilation
   d. Decelerating flow patterns cause poor oxygenation

3) Pplat pressures above _____ cause ventilator lung injury (VLI) and possible barotrauma?

   a. > 50 mmHg
   b. > 30 mmHg
   c. > 40 mmHg
   d. > 20 mmHg

4) Synchronized Intermittent Mandatory Ventilation (SIMV) is described as:

   a. Ventilator delivers breaths at a preset interval with spontaneous breathing allowed between ventilator-administered breaths
   b. Breaths are delivered at preset intervals, regardless of the patient's effort
   c. Ventilator delivers preset breaths in coordination with the respiratory effort of the patient. Spontaneous breathing is allowed between breaths.
   d. Volume targeted and pressure regulated

5) In volume control ventilation, it is most appropriate to monitor?

   a. PEEP
   b. PIP and V_t
   c. PIP, Pplat and static compliance
   d. Minute ventilation

6) You are transporting a 5kg, 3-day-old neonate in severe sepsis and metabolic acidosis who is intubated and sedated. The referring MD transitions care to you. What would be the most appropriate vent setting for this patient?

    a. SIMV 20, PC 20, V_{te} 30-40mL, PEEP 5, FiO_2 1.0
    b. SIMV 30, PC 10, V_{te} 30-40mL, PEEP 5, FiO_2 0.30
    c. SIMV 40, PC 10, V_{te} 20-30mL, PEEP 5, FiO_2 0.70
    d. SIMV 40, PC 12, V_{te} 15-30mL, PEEP 5, FiO_2 0.50

7) You are transporting a ventilated neonate who weighs 7kg with a current SpO_2 of 89%. The patient is sedated with diminished lung sounds bilaterally in the lower lobes. Current vent settings are: SIMV 24, PC 7, V_{te} 43 FiO_2 80%, PEEP 4. Which action is most appropriate?

    a. Increase inspiratory-to-expiratory (I:E) ratio
    b. Increase positive end-expiratory pressure (PEEP)
    c. Increase tidal volume (V_t)
    d. Increase respiratory rate (RR)

8) Your patient is demonstrating a sudden increase in PIP, however you also notice an elevated P_{plat}. The most likely cause would be?

    a. Acute respiratory distress syndrome (ARDS)
    b. COPD/Asthma
    c. Pulmonary hypertension
    d. Tension pneumothorax

9) Dead space is calculated by using which formula?

    a. 50% of V_t or approximately 4mL/kg
    b. 20% of V_t or approximately 1mL/kg
    c. 33% of V_t or approximately 1mL/1 pound of ideal body weight
    d. 7.5% of V_t or approximately 130mL

10) A 6-month-old, 12kg patient recently underwent surgery and has the following ABG: pH 7.42, $PaCO_2$ 38, PaO_2 52, HCO_3^- 25. Current ventilator settings: SIMV 24 V_{te} 68, f 32, PEEP 5, FiO_2 0.6. What adjustment to the current ventilator settings should be made?

    a. Increase FiO_2
    b. Increase PEEP
    c. Increase V_t
    d. Increase (f)

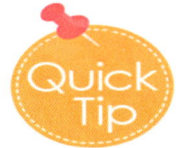

If you apply mechanical ventilation in the neonate, always use the lowest FiO_2 based on minutes after birth. This reduces the incidence of ductal closure and retinal detachment.

11) You are transporting a 3-year-old, 15kg patient involved in a MVC. Current vent settings: SIMV 20, V_t 60, FiO_2 1.0, PEEP 5, PIP 22, P_{plat} 19. ABG: pH 7.01, $PaCO_2$ 70, HCO_3^- 14, PaO_2 280, BE -8. What is your ABG interpretation?

    a. Mixed disturbance
    b. Respiratory acidosis
    c. Compensated respiratory acidosis
    d. Respiratory alkalosis

12) Pressure regulated volume control (PRVC) uses a combination of volume and pressure. How does this mode of ventilation accomplish this?

    a. Volume targeted
    b. Pressure targeted
    c. Volume targeted, pressure regulated
    d. Pressure targeted, volume driven

13) You have a 10-year-old asthmatic patient that is intubated for respiratory failure. What is the MOST appropriate I:E ratio setting?

    a. 1:2
    b. 1:1
    c. 3:1
    d. 1:4

Eric Bauer, MBA, FP-C, CCP-C, C-NPT

14) You are called to the scene of a motor vehicle collision (MVC). Your patient is an 8-year-old male who is immobilized and has obvious difficulty breathing. Assessment reveals circumoral cyanosis, diminished breath sounds throughout, and shallow chest expansion. SpO_2 is 89% on a NRB. Due to the patient's poor respiratory status, you and your partner have performed RSI, manually ventilated with 100% FiO_2, and continue fluid resuscitation. The patient is placed on your mechanical ventilator for the 40-minute flight. After approximately 10 minutes you note an increased PIP, decreasing chest expansion, and decreasing pulse oximetry. The most appropriate action is to:

a. Take the patient off the ventilator and manually ventilate the patient while confirming $EtCO_2$ waveform
b. Increase FiO_2 and PEEP
c. Switch to pressure control ventilation
d. Check the P_{plat} and if > 30 mmHg perform immediate chest decompression

15) When applying pressure support (PS) in a neonate on SIMV, what is the stopping point for allowing the spontaneous tidal volume?

a. Spontaneous breaths > 25% of controlled set V_t
b. Spontaneous breaths > 33% of controlled set V_t
c. Spontaneous breaths > 50% of controlled set V_t
d. Spontaneous breaths > 75% of controlled set V_t

16) Identify the medication with bronchodilating properties.

a. Etomidate
b. Ketamine
c. Atrovent
d. Versed

17) Your 30-week gestation neonate was born premature one day ago and has received surfactant replacement. What is a potential complication?

a. Increased functional residual capacity (FRC)
b. Shunt
c. Pulmonary hypertension
d. Air leak syndrome

18) Identify the following chest x-ray:

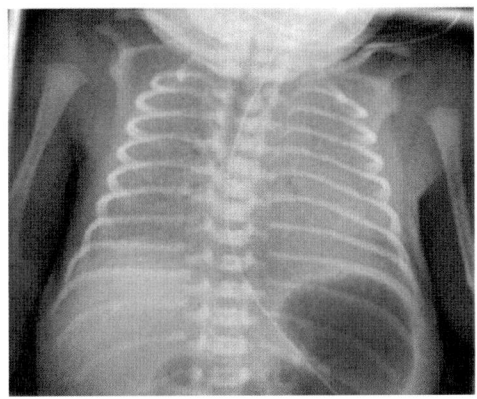

https://www.researchgate.net/figure/Acute-respiratory-distress-syndrome-with-widespread-ground-glass-opacity-and-air_fig1_50249686

a. Air leak syndrome
b. Hyaline membrane disease
c. Pulmonary hyperplasia
d. Neonatal congestive heart failure (CHF)

19) Identify the following chest x-ray:

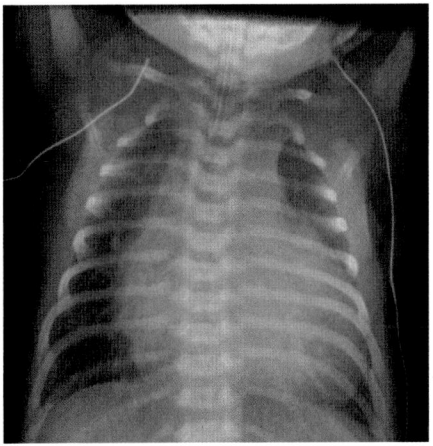

http://www.adhb.govt.nz/newborn/TeachingResources/Radiology/CXR/OtherCHF/NonstructuralCHF.jpg

a. Neonatal CHF
b. Air leak syndrome
c. Pulmonary hyperplasia
d. Diaphragmatic hernia

20) Identify the following chest x-ray:

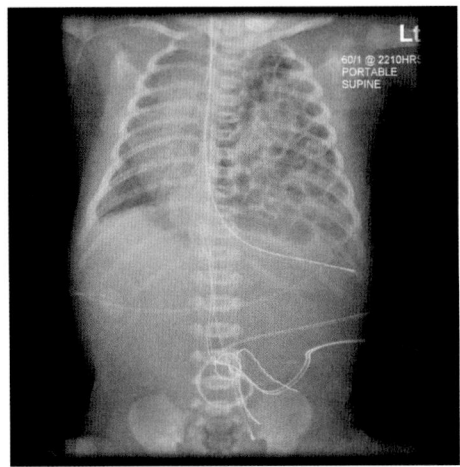

https://radiopaedia.org/cases/congenital-diaphragmatic-hernia

a. Pulmonary hypertension
b. Hemothorax
c. Diaphragmatic hernia
d. Pulmonary hyperplasia

21) Identify the following chest x-ray:

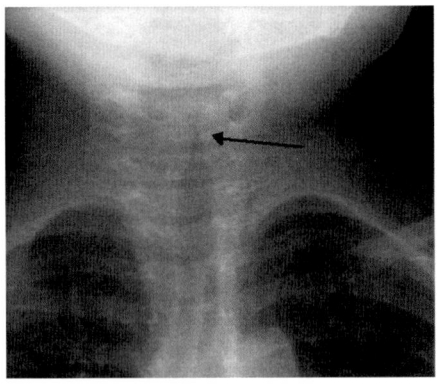

https://en.wikipedia.org/wiki/Steeple_sign

a. Epiglottitis
b. Croup
c. Air leak syndrome
d. Airway obstruction

22) Identify the following chest x-ray:

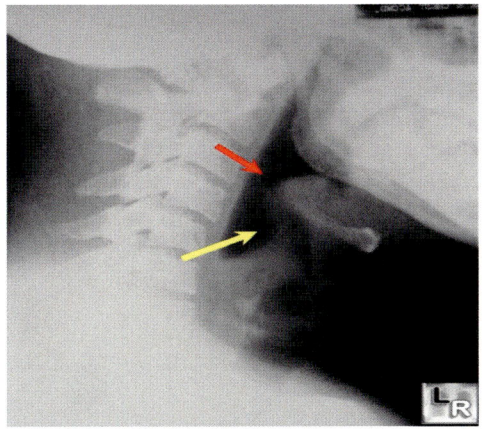

http://learningradiology.com/archives04/COW%20108-Epiglottitis/epiglottitiscorrect.htm

a. Airway obstruction
b. Croup
c. Epiglottitis
d. Air leak syndrome

23) Identify the following chest x-ray:

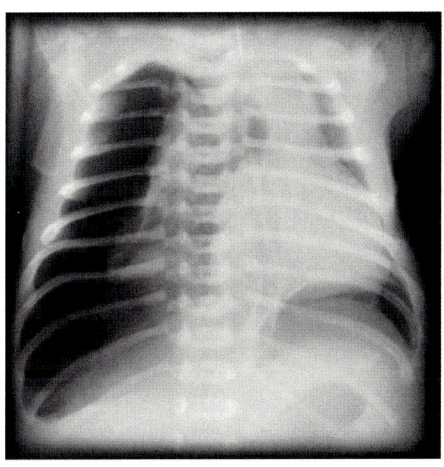

https://radiopaedia.org/articles/tension-pneumothorax

a. Croup
b. Hemothorax
c. Tension pneumothorax
d. Congestive heart failure (CHF)

Chapter 4 | Flight Physiology

1) You are flying at 45,000 feet mean sea level (MSL) and you experience an explosive decompression. How much time do you have to apply an O_2 source before you experience unconsciousness?

   a. 30-40 seconds
   b. 3-5 seconds
   c. 10-15 seconds
   d. 1 minute

2) Gay Lussac's law states that as you increase the temperature of a gas you would expect?

   a. An increase in pressure
   b. An increase in volume
   c. An increase in gas solubility
   d. A decrease in pressure

3) Dalton's law demonstrates that the concentration of O_2 at 18,000 ft. MSL is 21%. If the barometric pressure at 18,000 ft. MSL is 380 torr, what would the partial pressure of oxygen be at that altitude?

   a. 79 torr
   b. 14 torr
   c. 45 torr
   d. 34 torr

4) When administering high concentrations of oxygen to alleviate hypoxic hypoxia, you are altering which component of which gas law?

   a. Partial pressure; Boyle's law
   b. Partial pressure; Charles's law
   c. Solubility; Henry's law
   d. Solubility; Graham's law

5) An expanding endotracheal tube (ETT) in flight is an indication of what gas law?

   a. Henry's law
   b. Dalton's law
   c. Charles's law
   d. Boyle's law

6) Which statement best describes Henry's law?

   a. The sum of the partial pressures is equal to total atmospheric pressure
   b. The amount of gas in a solution is proportional to the partial pressure of gas above the solution
   c. The pressure of a gas is directly proportional to its temperature with the volume remaining constant
   d. At a constant temperature, a given volume of gas is inversely proportional to the pressure surrounding the gas

7) A patient suffering from decompression sickness is an example of which gas law?

   a. Boyle's law
   b. Graham's law
   c. Henry's law
   d. Dalton's law

8) Charles's law is best defined as:

   a. At a constant temperature, the pressure of a gas is inversely proportional to the volume of the gas
   b. The diffusion rate of a gas through a liquid medium is directly related to the solubility of the gas and is inversely proportional to the square root of its molecular weight
   c. At a constant pressure, the volume of a gas is very nearly proportional to its absolute temperature
   d. The amount of gas in a solution is proportional to the partial pressure of gas above the solution

9) For every 1000-feet increase in altitude, the ambient temperature will _____ an average of _____ Celsius.

   a. Decrease, 2°
   b. Increase, 1°
   c. Decrease, 4°
   d. Increase, 2°

10) While flying at cruising altitudes, the aspect of Boyle's law causes difficulty in controlling the rate of fluid drips. The most appropriate action would be to?

   a. Stop the IV fluids
   b. Place the fluid on a dial-a-flow
   c. Discontinue the IV bag
   d. Manually time the fluids with a pressure bag

FlightBridgeED, LLC

11) You are transporting a 4-year-old pediatric patient in respiratory distress via fixed wing aircraft. Their work of breathing has increased as you transition to level flight. According to Boyle's law, what intervention might improve their respiratory status?

      a. Intubation
      b. Nasal cannula @ 4 L/min
      c. Needle decompression
      d. Nasogastric tube placement

Chapter 5 | Little Tikes, Heat & Cold Injuries

1) With regards to a neonate, shivering is limited by?

    a. Cardiac output
    b. Muscle mass
    c. Glycogen stores
    d. Lactic acidosis

2) You are currently transferring a 3-year-old in severe hypothermia. Approximately 10 minutes out from the receiving facility the pediatric patient goes pulseless and apneic. Current esophageal temperature reads 28°C. You should withhold medications until the core temperature reaches?

    a. 29°C
    b. 30°C
    c. 32°C
    d. 34°C

3) You are called to transfer a 2-year-old due to seizure activity that started today. You note that the baby looks of normal weight and size. The father states his daughter drank one bottle of water this morning. You administer Valium and control the airway with intubation. How would you treat this patient?

Current labs are:

Na^+: 116	pH: 6.87
K^+: 2.5	$PaCO_2$: 112
Cl^-: 93	PaO_2: 130
BUN: 20	BE: -12
Cr: 0.9	SaO_2: 89%
Glu: 42	Serum osmolality: 310

What is your interpretation of the labs and current presentation?

4) In what order do you rewarm a hypothermic patient?

   a. Active external, passive external, active internal warming
   b. Passive external, active external, active internal warming
   c. Administer drugs and intubate
   d. Active passive, active internal & passive external warming

5) Temperature regulation in the neonate is limited by an immature hypothalamus and _____?

   a. Excessive glycogen stores
   b. Hypoactive thyroid
   c. Limited brown fat
   d. Small body surface area

6) Which of the following statements below is inaccurate regarding heat stroke?

   a. Respiratory alkalosis is a common finding in heat stroke
   b. Oxygen supply exceeds demand
   c. Level of consciousness is decreased
   d. Core temperature can exceed 104°F

7) A 2-year-old pediatric patient was left in a hot car. Resuscitation efforts have produced return of spontaneous circulation (ROSC). Which indicator would alert you to an associated diagnosis of rhabdomyolysis?

   a. Altered level of consciousness
   b. Elevated BUN
   c. Elevated creatine kinase (CK) levels
   d. Elevated troponin levels

8) You identify your 11-year-old patient is suffering from malignant hyperthermia. You know this is a result of what?

   a. Massive release of sodium
   b. Massive release of calcium
   c. Massive release of myoglobin
   d. Massive release of potassium

9) The primary treatment in reversing malignant hyperthermia is what medication?

   a. Vecuronium
   b. Fentanyl
   c. Methergine
   d. Dantrolene

10) A child that has sustained a salt-water drowning and aspirated approximately 4mL/kg of their body weight suffers from what?

   a. Hyperosmolar shift
   b. Hypo-osmolar shift
   c. Surfactant washout
   d. Absorption atelectasis

11) A 6-year-old presents to the ER straight from church camp. The referring RN states the child has diaphoresis, abdominal cramping with board like rigidity, tachycardia, hypertension, global weakness, nausea and vomiting. He states "I was bitten on the hand by a spider". Based on the presentation you suspect:

   a. Brown recluse spider envenomation
   b. Black widow spider envenomation
   c. Funnel web spider envenomation
   d. Tarantula spider envenomation

12) Management of the above patient after primary and secondary assessment has been completed would include all the following except?

   a. Tetanus immunization
   b. Fentanyl and Valium
   c. Skin testing and antivenin
   d. Magnesium sulfate administration

13) You are transferring an 8-year-old male patient that has suffered a snake bite of unknown species to the right calf. The snakebite happened approximately 45 minutes ago. What would be your best initial intervention?

   a. Apply ice and a restricting band above the bite site
   b. Immobilize and elevate the affected extremity
   c. Identify the snake species prior to starting any treatments
   d. Immobilize the affected extremity below the level of the heart

14) A 5-year-old pediatric patient was found down in the snow with a core temperature of 27°C. The following rhythm is identified, with no pulse present. Would you?

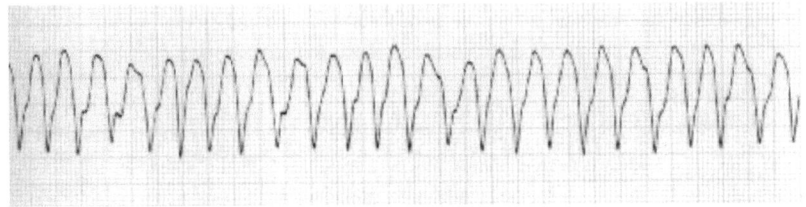

   a. Shock, CPR x2 minutes, shock
   b. Shock, wait until the core temperature is >30°C
   c. Shock, CPR x 2 minutes, Amiodarone
   d. CPR until the core temperature is >30°C, shock

Chapter 6 | Hematology & Electrolytes

1) Your main focus when treating a pediatric patient in DIC is to:

   a. Administer heparin
   b. Administer fresh frozen plasma (FFP)
   c. Correct the underlying pathology
   d. Replacement of clotting factors

2) You have administered 2 units of PRBCs. Your patient's initial hemoglobin and hematocrit (H&H) was 6 and 18. You would expect their H&H to increase to:

   a. 10 and 22
   b. 8 and 20
   c. 8 and 24
   d. 9 and 21

3) Your 1-year-old pediatric patient is currently receiving a magnesium infusion due to hypomagnesemia (1.2 mEq/L initially). Upon assessment, which finding would alert you to immediately stop the infusion?

   a. An increase in the blood pressure of 15 mmHg
   b. Occasional PVCs on the ECG
   c. Absent patellar reflexes
   d. Diarrhea

4) You are treating a 12-year-old patient in diabetic ketoacidosis (DKA) with a potassium level of 3.1 mEq/L. When looking at their ECG, what would you expect to find?

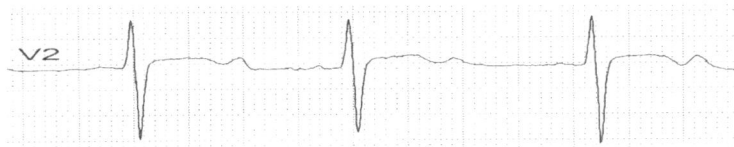

   a. ST segment elevation
   b. Peaked T waves
   c. U waves
   d. Increased PR intervals

5) Your 15-year-old patient has a history of hypoparathyrioidism. They are currently complaining of numbness and tingling around the mouth and in their toes. You would anticipate which abnormal electrolyte finding?

    a. Hyperkalemia
    b. Hypocalcemia
    c. Hyponatremia
    d. Hypermagnesemia

6) Alice is an 8-year-old female. Her current hematocrit (Hct) is 58% and serum Na^+ is 156 mEq/L. What is the most likely cause of these findings?

    a. Acute renal failure
    b. Dehydration
    c. Fluid overload
    d. Normal finding in a pediatric patient

7) You are transporting a 1 month-old infant with a diagnosis of CHF and pulmonary hypertension who has been receiving high doses of Lasix. On assessment, you notice generalized muscle weakness, flat neck veins and diminished deep tendon reflexes (DTRs). You suspect hyponatremia. What other assessment findings would help you confirm this diagnosis?

    a. Abdominal distension
    b. Dry mucous membranes
    c. Oliguria
    d. Increased specific gravity of urine

8) DIC is a primary problem with?

    a. Bleeding
    b. Platelet function failure
    c. Clotting
    d. Deactivation of thrombin

9) You are transporting a 15-year-old patient involved in a traumatic resuscitation. They have received 5 units of PRBCs rapidly. What should you be considering in this patient?

    a. Fluid overload
    b. Citrate toxicity
    c. Hemolytic reaction
    d. Methemoglobinemia

10) How would you manage the aforementioned patient?

   a. Calcium administration
   b. Benadryl administration
   c. Lasix administration
   d. Methylene blue administration

11) You are called to transport a 16-year-old who sustained multiple gunshot wounds during a gang-related activity. You are told that the patient required multiple units of PRBCs due to the amount of blood loss from the wounds. You anticipate monitoring the patient's ECG closely for changes indicating what?

   a. Hypernatremia
   b. Hypercalcemia
   c. Hyperkalemia
   d. Hypermagnesemia

12) An 8-year-old male is diagnosed with acute cardiac collapse secondary to myocarditis. Upon assessment, you note the following: BP 72/38, HR 128, RR 34, urine output of 30 mL over the past 3 hours, CVP 12mmHg, PAP 32/26mmHg, PCWP 23mmHg, CI 1.7 L/min/m2. When evaluating this patient's glomerular filtration rate (GFR), what laboratory value would be best to look at?

   a. Serum creatinine
   b. Urinalysis
   c. BUN
   d. Urine creatinine clearance

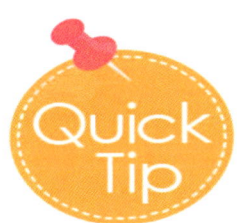

**In the pediatric population, with severe anemia (hemoglobin <5 g/dL) not secondary to acute hemorrhage, PRBCs should be administered in the amount/kg equal to the laboratory value of the hemoglobin.
Transfuse:**

**3 mL/kg for a hemoglobin of 3 g/dL
4 mL/kg for a hemoglobin of 4 g/dL
5 mL/kg for a hemoglobin of 5 g/dL**

Subsequent transfusions are administered at 10-15 mL/kg to avoid heart failure.

Madden M (2013). *Pediatric Fundamental of Critical Care Support*; (2nd Ed)

13) A 6-year-old pediatric patient is being transferred to a level 1 pediatric ICU after sustaining a venomous snake bite approximately 6 hours ago. They are having bleeding from their IV site as well as the initial wound. You notice the referring facility has marked the area of edema and written the time in the area. Which of the following lab values would be suggestive of DIC?

    a. Decreased platelets, increased fibrinogen, normal PT/PTT, normal thrombin time
    b. Decreased platelets, decreased fibrinogen, prolonged PT/PTT, prolonged thrombin time
    c. Increased platelets, increased fibrinogen, normal PT/PTT, normal thrombin time
    d. Increased platelets, decreased fibrinogen, prolonged PT/PTT, prolonged thrombin time

14) The following calculation $[Na^+ - (Cl^- + HCO_3^-) + K^+]$ represents?

    a. Strong acids
    b. Corrected anion gap
    c. Cations
    d. Uncorrected anion gap

15) Fluid loss in a dehydrated patient will most critically increase serum levels of which of the following?

    a. Sodium
    b. Calcium
    c. Potassium
    d. Chloride

16) What is the classic sign of hypocalcemia?

    a. Kehr's sign
    b. Grey-Turner's sign
    c. Trousseau's sign
    d. Brudzinski's sign

17) All of the following are triggers for sickle cell crisis except?

    a. Stress
    b. Cold weather
    c. Poor fluid intake
    d. Altitude changes

Chapter 7 | Little Hearts – RPMs & PUMP

1) **Practice**
   - CVP 1
   - CI 1.8
   - PA S/D 11/5
   - PCWP 4
   - SVR 1800

   - Identify the underlying presentation.

     a. Hypovolemic shock
     b. Left systolic dysfunction
     c. Neurogenic shock
     d. Septic shock

2) **Practice**
   - CVP 16
   - CI 1.3
   - PA S/D 44/26
   - PCWP 27
   - SVR 2052

   - Identify the underlying presentation.

     a. Hypovolemic shock
     b. Left systolic dysfunction
     c. Neurogenic shock
     d. Obstructive shock

3) **Practice**
   - CVP 0
   - CI 6.1
   - PA S/D 30/14
   - PCWP 6
   - SVR 400

   Identify the underlying presentation.

     a. Right side heart failure
     b. Cardiogenic shock
     c. Neurogenic shock
     d. Septic shock

4) **Practice**
   - CVP 1
   - CI 1.6
   - PA S/D 12/8
   - PCWP 5
   - SVR 300

Identify the underlying presentation.

   a. Hypovolemic shock
   b. Left systolic dysfunction
   c. Neurogenic shock
   d. Septic shock

5) Your patient is experiencing left ventricular diastolic failure. What would your first line therapy be focused on?

   a. Augmentation of left ventricular clearing
   b. Increasing preload
   c. Increasing afterload
   d. Decreasing preload

6) Pulmonary capillary wedge pressure (PCWP) represents?

   a. Afterload of the heart
   b. Right sided preload
   c. Right sided ventricular pressure
   d. Directly reflects left atrial pressure

7) When obtaining a PCWP on your cardiac patient you note a large V wave on the waveform. After confirming that the PA catheter is correctly placed and the balloon is not ruptured, what condition do you suspect?

   a. Tricuspid valve regurgitation
   b. Pulmonic valve stenosis
   c. Aortic valve stenosis
   d. Mitral valve regurgitation

8) The dicrotic notch on the arterial waveform of a Swan-Ganz catheter is reflective of what mechanical event in the heart?

   a. Tricuspid valve closure
   b. Pulmonic valve closure
   c. Mitral valve closure
   d. Aortic valve closure

9) A normal CVP/RAP reading would be?

   a. 6-10mmHg
   b. 2-6mmHg
   c. 12-16mmHg
   d. 22-28mmHg

10) You note the following hemodynamic parameters on your neonate: CVP 2, PCWP 12, CI 1.5, SVR 1800. What is your clinical diagnosis?

   a. Cardiogenic shock
   b. Hypovolemic shock
   c. Neurogenic shock
   d. Sepsis

11) The central line readings obtained in the neonatal ICU prior to transport of a 2-week neonate with an outflow obstruction heart defect are as follows: CVP 13, CI 1.4, and PCWP 18. This could indicate what problem for the patient?

   a. Hypovolemic shock
   b. Septic shock
   c. Cardiogenic shock
   d. Anaphylactic shock

12) What is a normal systemic vascular resistance (SVR) measurement?

   a. 200-400 dyne-sec/cm^{-5}
   b. 400-1000 dyne-sec/cm^{-5}
   c. 800-1200 dyne-sec/cm^{-5}
   d. 1200-1800 dyne-sec/cm^{-5}

13) Cardiac output determined by?

   a. CO = SV x HR
   b. CO = MAP – HR
   c. CO = BP x HR
   d. CO = MAP / HR

14) Mean arterial pressure (MAP) is calculated by?

   a. MAP = (HR + DBP) / 2
   b. MAP = [(SBP + (2 x DBP) / 3]
   c. MAP = [SBP + (2 x DBP) / 2]
   d. MAP = [SBP + (3 x DBP) / 2]

15) The _____ measures filling pressures on the right side of the heart as the tip lies in the right atrium.

   a. Pulmonary capillary wedge pressure (PCWP)
   b. Central venous pressure (CVP)
   c. End left diastolic pressure
   d. Right ventricular (RV) pressure

16) The normal SvO$_2$ (central venous oxygen) concentration is?

   a. 70-90%
   b. 50-60%
   c. 30-60%
   d. 60-80%

17) The normal range for a PCWP is?

   a. 4-9mmHg
   b. 6-10mmHg
   c. 8-12mmHg
   d. 12-15mmHg

18) Which of the following pulmonary artery pressures are within normal limits.

   a. PAP 34/24, PCWP 12
   b. PAP 30/20, PCWP 10
   c. PAP 28/18, PCWP 20
   d. PAP 24/14, PCWP 12

19) While transferring a patient out of the pediatric ICU, you note the patient's current hemodynamic parameters. Their current CI is 1.6, CVP 17, PAP 44/22 mmHg, and PCWP 18 with a current BP of 78/60 and HR of 120. These hemodynamic parameters would suggest what diagnosis?

a. Neurogenic shock
b. Right ventricular infarction
c. Septic shock
d. Cardiogenic shock

20) The central venous pressure (CVP) monitors what?

a. Intra-arterial pressure
b. Pulmonary artery pressure
c. Right atrial pressure
d. Femoral venous pressure

21) Common causes of elevated pulmonary artery (PA) pressures encompass all the following except?

a. Left ventricular failure
b. Mitral valve stenosis
c. Mitral valve regurgitation
d. Tricuspid valve regurgitation

22) The central line reading obtained in the pediatric ICU shows: CVP 8, CI 1.4, and PCWP 13. This could indicate what problem for the patient?

a. Hypovolemia
b. Heart failure
c. Anaphylactic shock
d. Septic shock

23) When transporting and assessing a patient with a pulmonary catheter, if the PAP is more than 5mmHg above the PCWP, it signals which abnormal condition?

a. High SVR
b. Pulmonary hypertension
c. Left ventricular failure
d. Mitral valve insufficiency

24) Which type of medication blocks the renin-angiotensin-aldosterone (RAA) system to help with heart failure?

a. Beta-blocker
b. Calcium-channel blockers
c. Angiotensin-converting enzyme (ACE) inhibitors
d. Thiazide diuretics

25) _____ is a drug that has potent alpha effects used to increase SVR in profound vasodilatory redistributive shock states such as sepsis and neurogenic shock.

a. Dopamine
b. Esmolol
c. Nipride
d. Neo-synephrine

26) A neonate has sudden decompensation two days after going home with parents. The infant was full-term and seemingly healthy. On assessment you note pre-ductal SpO_2 on right hand of 90% and identify lower extremity SpO_2 at 70%. No femoral pulses are noted and you find a distended abdomen. What is your clinical diagnosis?

a. Acyanotic heart defect
b. Atrial Septal defect
c. Left outflow obstruction defect
d. Ventral Septal defect

27) Infants are born with _____ axis deviation?

a. Normal
b. Right
c. Left
d. Extreme right

28) You note left axis deviation on your EKG for a 1-hour-old neonate. This would indicate?

a. Normal findings
b. Acyanotic heart defect
c. Left ventricular hypertrophy
d. Right ventricular hypertrophy

29) Your neonate has an order for continuous prostaglandin administration. What is the starting dose?

   a. 0.01-0.5 mcg/kg/min
   b. 0.05-0.1 mcg/kg/min
   c. 1.0-1.5 mcg/kg/min
   d. 1.5-2 mcg/kg/min

30) You are called to transfer a 5-month-old infant with Tetralogy of Fallot with DiGeorge syndrome. You know this patient could have episodes of seizure activity secondary to?

   a. Hyponatremia
   b. Hypoglycemia
   c. Hypomagnesemia
   d. Hypocalcemia

31) Dopamine's alpha-adrenergic effects are related to?

   a. Decreased renal vascular resistance
   b. Dilation of peripheral vascular resistance
   c. Coronary vasoconstriction
   d. Beta-1 peripheral vascular resistance

32) Which medication causes decreased pulmonary vascular resistance?

   a. Dopamine
   b. Levophed
   c. Nitroprusside
   d. Norepinephrine

Chapter 8 | Endocrine & Renal – Hormones & Pee

1) Your teenage DKA patient is being treated with insulin and fluid replacement. You note a decrease in mental status with associated lethargy and their GCS is now 7. This would most likely indicate?

   a. Cerebral edema
   b. Acute stroke
   c. Hyponatremia
   d. Diabetes Insipidus

2) You are requested to transport a 12-year-old diagnosed with DKA. They are 5'4" and weigh 56kg. While in the ED, they have been breathing at a rate of 38 breaths per minute and you notice upon assessment that the patient appears fatigued. You make the decision to intubate the patient and request current ABGs. They are as follows: pH 7.01, $PaCO_2$ 23, PaO_2 280, HCO_3^- 17. She is currently on a NRB at 15LPM. Which of the following plans would best suit this patient initially?

   a. Continue paralysis and sedation after intubation and set vent to: SIMV 12, Vt 870, FiO_2 0.6, PEEP 5
   b. Continue paralysis and sedation after intubation and set vent to: AC 12, Vt 600, FiO_2 0.7, PEEP 5
   c. Continue sedation after intubation and set vent to: AC 30, Vt 850, FiO_2 0.7, PEEP 5
   d. Continue sedation after intubation and set vent to: SIMV 30, Vt 500, FiO_2 0.6, PEEP 5

3) Regarding your patient above, treatment surrounding dropping glucose is based on the following protocol?

   a. Glucose decrease < 200 mg/dL per hour
   b. Glucose decrease < 100 mg/dL per hour
   c. Glucose decrease > 200 mg/dL per hour
   d. Glucose decrease > 100 mg/dL per hour

4) Your 3-year-old male patient has sustained traumatic injuries after being involved in an MVC. He has become hypovolemic and is demonstrating signs of shock. Which of the following would you also anticipate along with this?

   a. Pre-renal failure
   b. Renal failure
   c. Post-renal failure

d. Chronic Renal Failure

5) You are called to transport a 6-year-old patient in DKA. Which of the following assessment findings would indicate that this patient's DKA is deteriorating?

    a. Urine pH less than 5.8
    b. An increase in bicarb from 22 mEq/L to 25 mEq/L
    c. Deep tendon reflexes (DTRs) decreasing from +2 to +1
    d. Potassium levels decreasing from 6.3 mEq/L to 5.2 mEq/L

6) Which would be the best choice to treat diabetes insipidus (DI)?

    a. Aggressive correction of acidosis using bicarbonate administration and respiratory compensation
    b. Aggressive glucose control with insulin
    c. Aggressive fluid management with DDAVP
    d. Aggressive diuresis using diuretics

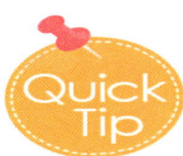

Diabetes insipidus is caused by a deficiency of vasopressin or resistance of the kidneys to vasopressin. Vasopressin is also known as anti-diuretic hormone (ADH). This causes excessive urination and hypernatremia. Treatment includes administration of desmopressin (DDAVP). DDAVP is a synthetic form of vasopressin. It works on the kidneys to help decrease the amount of urine produced.

7) During treatment of pediatric DKA, at what glucose level would you start a dextrose maintenance infusion?

    a. 100-150 mg/dL
    b. 150-200 mg/dL
    c. 200-250 mg/dL
    d. 250-300 mg/dL

8) A 2-year-old presents with fever, hyperglycemia and lethargy for the past 3 hours. Vital signs: BP 72/42, HR 146, and RR 32. Upon assessment, you note dry mucous membranes and capillary refill of 4 seconds. Current labs are: K^+ 3.0 mEq/L, glucose 485 mg/dL. ABGs: pH 7.1, $PaCO_2$ 22, HCO_3^- 17, PaO_2 98. Which of the following types of fluids is most appropriate initially for this patient?

    a. Lactated Ringers (LR)
    b. Normal saline (0.9%)
    c. ½ Normal saline (0.45%)
    d. Hypertonic saline (3%)

9) Which of the following laboratory findings would you expect to see in a patient with a diagnosis of syndrome of inappropriate anti-diuretic hormone (SIADH)?

   a. Hypoglycemia
   b. Dilutional hyponatremia
   c. Hyperkalemia
   d. Dilutional hypercalcemia

10) What is the leading cause of neonatal sepsis?

   a. Pneumonia
   b. Low birth weight
   c. Group B strep
   d. Hyaline membrane disease

11) Which lab finding would be most associated with diabetes insipidus?

   a. Elevated capillary blood glucose
   b. Relative hyperkalemia
   c. Relative hypocalcemia
   d. Urinary hypo-osmolality

12) A key component used in the management of both DKA and HHNK in the pediatric population is?

   a. Aggressive fluid resuscitation
   b. Rapid correction of the high glucose
   c. Aggressive correction of the metabolic acidosis
   d. Aggressive correction of the associated hyperkalemia

13) Systemic inflammatory response syndrome (SIRS) can lead to multi-organ dysfunction. Which of the following organs is involved first?

   a. Brain
   b. Liver
   c. Lungs
   d. Heart

14) You are treating a 15-year-old who is very lethargic and only responsive to painful stimuli. They have a history of type I diabetes mellitus and have been sick with a virus for the past couple of days. When reviewing lab results, what would you expect to find initially?

    a. Hyperglycemia, hypokalemia, acidosis, elevated serum osmolality
    b. Hyperglycemia, hyperkalemia, acidosis, elevated serum osmolality
    c. Hyperglycemia, hypokalemia, alkalosis, elevated serum osmolality
    d. Hyperglycemia, hyperkalemia, alkalosis, elevated serum osmolality

15) You are transferring a 5-year-old pediatric patient with a recent craniotomy to remove a tumor. They are currently awake, alert and answering your questions appropriately. There are no signs of any neurological deficits. Vitals are currently: BP 112/76, HR 88, RR 22, SpO_2 97% on 2L NC, glucose 96 mg/dL. Since the craniotomy, they have been urinating approximately 50 mL/hr. Within the last couple of hours, urine output has increased to 350 mL/hr and has a specific gravity of 1.001. What would you suspect?

    a. Development of type 2 diabetes mellitus
    b. Diabetes insipidus
    c. Syndrome of inappropriate anti-diuretic hormone (SIADH)
    d. Hypervolemia

16) Based upon the diagnosis of your 5-year-old pediatric patient from above, what lab findings would you anticipate?

    a. Oliguria, high serum osmolality, hypernatremia, and low urine specific gravity
    b. Oliguria, low serum osmolality, hyponatremia, and high urine specific gravity
    c. Polyuria, high serum osmolality, hypernatremia, and low urine specific gravity
    d. Polyuria, low serum osmolality, hyponatremia, and high urine specific gravity

17) You have a 13-year-old patient with a history of insulin dependent diabetes. They are admitted to the local ICU. Family states that they have had a cold over the past week and have become lethargic over the last 24 hours. Lab results are as follows: Na⁺ 150, Cl⁻ 103, glucose 504, WBC 12.3, bands 14%, leukocytes represent 68%. The most likely cause of this patient's DKA is:

    a. Acute infection
    b. Dehydration
    c. Noncompliance with insulin
    d. Pancreatitis

18) Black and blue ecchymosis around the umbilicus is called?

    a. Kehr's sign
    b. Cullen's sign
    c. McBurney's point
    d. Grey-Turners sign

19) The drug of choice for treating seizures in the pediatric population is:

    a. Luminal
    b. Phenytoin
    c. Ativan
    d. Glycopyrrolate

20) When treating a pediatric patient with suspected DKA, what values would you use to differentiate the diagnosis of DKA from hyperosmolar hyperglycemic nonketotic (HHNK) condition?

    a. A serum glucose of 550 mg/dL
    b. A serum potassium of 3.5 mEq/L
    c. Positive serum ketones
    d. A serum osmolality of 320 mOsm/L

Chapter 9 | Trauma – Trips, Spills, Breaks & Catastrophes

1) Beck's triad has all of the following EXCEPT?

    a. Jugular venous distention (JVD)
    b. Muffled heart tones
    c. Left shoulder pain
    d. Narrowing pulse pressures

2) The consensus formula calculates hourly fluid replacement for pediatric burn patients. What equation would you use?

    a. 2mL x kg x % BSA
    b. 3mL x kg x % BSA
    c. 4mL x kg x % BSA
    d. 5mL x kg x % BSA

3) Minimum urine output for the pediatric burn patient with non-suspected rhabdomyolysis would be?

    a. 0.5-1mL/kg/hr
    b. 1-2mL/kg/hr
    c. 3-5mL/kg/hr
    d. 6-8mL/kg/hr

4) You have a 7kg female patient involved in an MVC that caught fire. She has received first-degree burns to her abdomen and lower back, and second and third degree burns to her face, head and both arms. What percentage would you calculate her total body surface area (BSA) burns as?

    a. 27%
    b. 32%
    c. 36%
    d. 63%

5) You are caring for a pediatric burn patient weighing 20kg with 45% BSA of second and third-degree burns, with time of injury at 2 hours ago. The referring facility states they've given 300mL LR thus far. Using the consensus formula, what would your fluid resuscitation amount be for the first 8 hours taking into account volume already administered?

    a. 1,050mL; 175mL/hr
    b. 1,350mL; 169mL/hr
    c. 1,400mL; 180mL/hr
    d. 1,800mL; 200mL/hr

6) Which of the following is not a treatment strategy when dealing with rhabdomyolosis and myoglobinuria?

   a. Mannitol
   b. Sodium bicarbonate (NaHCO3⁻) treatment
   c. Fluid resuscitation
   d. Vasopressin administration

7) The most likely secondary complication associated with a pediatric patient that has suffered a pelvic fracture is?

   a. Renal artery laceration
   b. Intestinal perforation
   c. Bladder injury
   d. Retroperitoneal hemorrhage

8) You are called for a 20kg pediatric burn patient that has 45% second and third-degree burns. The patient was burned approximately 26 hours ago. The physician reports that the patient has had a total of 3 liters of fluid in a 24-hour period because he does not want the patient to get cerebral edema. Using the consensus formula, how much fluid should this pediatric patient have received in the first 24 hours of burn care?

   a. 1,350 mL
   b. 1,800 mL
   c. 2,700 mL
   d. 3,600 mL

9) During transport of a 14-year-old burn patient, you notice an absent P wave and an increased QRS interval on the ECG. Initial ECG showed sinus tachycardia (ST) in the 160s with peaked T waves. What electrolyte abnormality do you suspect?

   a. Hypomagnesemia
   b. Hyperkalemia
   c. Hypercalcemia
   d. Hypokalemia

10) You are taking care of a 5-year-old pediatric patient with a left lower leg fracture. The leg has been splinted but not straightened. The child is now screaming with pain every time you try to do an assessment. What is your first action prior to transport?

   a. Straighten the fracture
   b. Pain medication and secondary assessment

c. Administer sedation
d. Transport with leg splinted in current position

11) You are called to the scene of an MVC involving a semi-truck versus a car. On arrival, you find a 16-year-old male patient in the front seat with agonal respirations. Prior to extrication, the patient becomes pulseless and apneic. The most common cause of mortality with this type of accident is an aortic tear. An aortic tear is commonly associated with which of the following?

    a. Blunt force injury to the chest wall
    b. Penetration injury to the chest wall
    c. Acceleration/deceleration injury
    d. Cardiac contusion

12) Sudden cardiac death associated with high-speed projectile objects are described as commotio cordis. This is a result of which of the following?

    a. Cardiac tamponade
    b. Cardiac contusion
    c. Fatal dysrhythmia
    d. Aortic arch tear

13) You are caring for an 8-year-old with an orbital wall and floor fracture. You know this type of injury may cause?

    a. Optic nerve compression
    b. Ptosis
    c. Entrapment of intraocular muscles
    d. Nystagmus

14) Intraosseous (IO) access is contraindicated with?

    a. PRBC administration
    b. Gestational age < 36 weeks
    c. Previous failed attempt in extremity
    d. Rhabdomyolysis

15) You are transporting a 13-year-old obese child who complains of right knee pain. No injury event is reported and the pain has been ongoing for 3 months. What is the likely cause?

    a. Fibromyalgia
    b. Normal growth pain
    c. Slipped capital femoral epiphysis
    d. Femoral vein thrombosis

16) You are called to transfer a 4-year-old that was found unresponsive in a hot car. The child is hyperthermic with a core temperature of 104°F. The hallmark indicator that rhabdomyolysis is occurring is?

    a. Altered mental status
    b. Increased BUN
    c. Hyperthermia
    d. Elevated creatine kinase (CK)

17) A 15-year-old trauma patient from the emergency department undergoes fluid resuscitation with 3L of normal saline solution and 4 units of unwarmed packed red blood cells. They remain unconscious, intubated, and ventilated with 100% oxygen. They have received sedation and remain immobilized on a backboard. You should remain concerned about:

    a. Decreased clotting times due to the banked PRBC's
    b. Alkalosis due to the blood administration
    c. Hypothermia due to unwarmed blood
    d. Hypokalemia due to the blood administration

18) You are on the scene of a 15-year-old patient who sustained a gunshot wound to the left chest. The left chest has been decompressed with a needle. The patient is intubated and continues to desaturate and you note an increase in subcutaneous air. How will you manage this patient?

    a. Re-needle the left chest
    b. Advance the ETT below the level of the injury
    c. Insert a chest tube
    d. Decrease the respiratory rate down to 10 breaths per minute

19) Myoglobinuria, if left untreated, will result in what critical condition?

    a. Hyperkalemic crisis
    b. Acute tubular necrosis
    c. Cardiomyopathy
    d. Polycystic kidney disease

20) When administering PRBC's, you can expect a rise in hemoglobin (Hgb) and hematocrit (Hct) of _____ for each unit of blood?

    a. 1gm/dL increase in the hemoglobin and 3% increase in the hematocrit
    b. 2gm/dL increase in the hemoglobin and a 3% increase in the hematocrit
    c. 1gm/dL increase in the hemoglobin and a 5% increase in the hematocrit

d. 2gm/dL increase in the hemoglobin and a 5% increase in the hematocrit

21) You are dispatched for a transfer to a level 1 trauma center for a 16-year-old with massive head, chest and abdominal trauma from an MVC. They have received 5 units of PRBCs prior to your arrival. They continue to bleed profusely from all wounds despite direct pressure to control bleeding. You suspect DIC. What treatment do you expect to administer?

   a. Dobutamine
   b. PRBCs
   c. Rapid fluid volume replacement
   d. Platelets, cryoprecipitate, and FFP

22) You respond to a rural facility to transport a 12-year-old patient with head, chest and thoracic spine trauma. Upon viewing the X-ray, you note a widened mediastinum, obliteration of the aortic knob and the presence of a pleural cap. You suspect what injury?

   a. Tension pneumothorax
   b. Esophageal disruption
   c. Aortic disruption
   d. Tracheal bronchial disruption

23) How much circulating blood volume does your pediatric patient have?

   a. 55-60 mL/kg
   b. 65-70 mL/kg
   c. 75-80 mL/kg
   d. 85-90 mL/kg

24) You are transferring a 5-year-old pediatric trauma patient for emergent abdominal surgery. Which of the following would be considered an EMTALA violation?

   a. No transferring physician's signature
   b. Transfer from a pediatric ICU
   c. Medical records are transferred with the patient
   d. Receiving physician accepts transfer of the patient

25) Fractures of the 1st-3rd ribs should indicate a high index of suspicion for which injury?

   a. Esophageal rupture
   b. Aortic dissection
   c. Pulmonary contusion
   d. Liver laceration

26) When inserting a chest tube, the correct insertion site recommended is?

   a. 3rd intercostal space (ICS) mid-clavicular
   b. 3rd ICS between mid-axillary and anterior axillary
   c. 5th ICS mid-clavicular
   d. 5th ICS between mid-axillary and anterior axillary

27) You arrive on the scene to manage a 10-year-old fall victim. Vital signs are: BP 70/32, HR 60, RR 30, SpO$_2$ 94%. EMS reports the patient had a brief loss of consciousness, but now has a GCS of 14. You note a deformity to the right femur and they are complaining of neck pain. Your diagnosis of this patient is?

   a. Epidural bleed
   b. Hypovolemic shock
   c. Neurogenic shock
   d. Subdural bleed

28) A patient presenting with Beck's triad is most likely experiencing:

   a. Liver laceration
   b. Tension pneumothorax
   c. Increased ICP
   d. Cardiac tamponade

29) Injury patterns associated with rear impact collisions are?

   a. T12-L1 and C-spine fractures
   b. Clavicle, ribs, femur, tib/fib injuries and abdominal injuries
   c. T-spine fractures, clavicle and pelvic fractures
   d. Fractured ribs, skull fractures, patella, femur, acetabular fractures and dislocated hip

30) You are called to transfer an 8-year-old patient that was involved in a head-on accident with a semi-truck. The patient is currently showing clinical signs of hypoxia with a NRB at 15 L/min being administered. Currently the patient has a GCS of 10 and breathing shallow and rapid at 28 breaths per minute. Vital signs are: BP 100/70, HR 139, RR 28. Skin is pale, dry and warm. Labs: H&H 7&19. The patient has a current urine output of 0.5mL/kg/hr for the past 3 hours. What type of shock is the patient suffering from?

   a. Hypoxic hypoxia
   b. Stagnant hypoxia
   c. Hypemic hypoxia

d. Histotoxic hypoxia

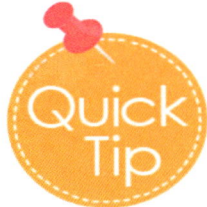

Fluid maintenance in the neonate is significantly different in comparison to pediatrics. The standard 4-2-1 rule doesn't apply. Instead, for any neonate >28 weeks gestation, start with a maintenance of 100cc/kg/day of D10.

In addition, a glucose infusion rate (GIR) can be titrated to be more specific with rate of infusion and dextrose concentration, never to exceed D12. The standard GIR infusion is 6-8mg/kg/day. This is an essential part of neonatal resuscitation, with emphasis on strict glucose control and constant evaluation of dextrose percentage, due to its effects on the neonatal brain.

Referenced from: http://www.openanesthesia.org/fluid-management/

Chapter 10 | Neurological Emergencies

1) Your patient has the following hemodynamic parameters: BP 90/60, HR 110, RR 22 & irregular, ICP 29, CVP 20, PA 32/14, PCWP 15. Identify the cerebral perfusion pressure (CPP)?

   a. 41
   b. 52
   c. 87
   d. 81

2) Based on the question above, what is the target CPP for the pediatric patient?

   a. 50 mmHg
   b. 60 mmHg
   c. 70 mmHg
   d. 80 mmHg

3) You respond for a 10-year-old that fell at school. On arrival, you find your patient with an altered level of consciousness. EMS states that they had a brief loss of consciousness and a period of lucidness prior to the current decline in GCS. This presentation most often presents with what type of head trauma?

   a. Epidural bleed
   b. Intraventricular bleed
   c. Subdural bleed
   d. Diffuse axonal injury

4) Cushing's triad consists of?

   a. Widening pulse pressures, tachycardia and normal respirations
   b. Hypertension, bradycardia and respiratory changes (Cheyne-Stokes)
   c. Hypotension, widening pulse pressures and bradycardia
   d. Hypertension, tachycardia and narrowing pulse pressures

5) Diffuse axonal injury will most likely represent how on a CT scan?

   a. Normal and unidentifiable
   b. Granulated or salt and pepper appearance
   c. Identified by cervical spine subluxation
   d. Petechial hemorrhages throughout

6) Your patient has an ICP of 25. Their current BP is 100/60. Their cerebral perfusion pressure is approximately?

   a. 45 mmHg
   b. 48 mmHg
   c. 72 mmHg
   d. 82 mmHg

7) You respond to a rural facility to pick up a pediatric patient with a diagnosis of a skull fracture. Upon arrival, the x-ray shows multiple fractures that radiate from a compressed area. What type of skull fracture does this patient have?

   a. Basilar fracture
   b. Linear stellate fracture
   c. Diastatic fracture
   d. Depressed fracture

8) The classic description of a patient suffering from an epidural bleed is?

   a. Rapid onset of unconsciousness, posturing and seizures
   b. Unconsciousness, followed by a brief period of lucidity and a period of rapid decrease in the level of consciousness
   c. Slow loss of consciousness, pupillary changes, and seizures
   d. Slow loss of consciousness, ipsilateral posturing and contralateral pupillary changes

9) A basilar skull fracture is associated with all of the following EXCEPT:

   a. CSF rhinorrhea
   b. CSF otorrhea
   c. Seventh cranial nerve palsy
   d. Eleventh cranial nerve paralysis

10) When monitoring invasive intracranial pressure lines, the transducer should be leveled at the?

   a. Foramen of Kellie
   b. Foramen of Ovale
   c. Foramen of Monro
   d. Foramen of Magnum

11) A 16-year-old patient is diagnosed with Brown-Sequard Syndrome. Brown-Sequard Syndrome presents with which of the following signs/symptoms?

   a. Complete flaccidity below the level of the injury
   b. Ipsilateral motor loss, contralateral pain loss

c. Greater weakness in upper extremities than in lower extremities
d. Complete motor, pain and temperature loss below the level of the injury

12) A 15-year-old has a diagnosis of subarachnoid hemorrhage (SAH) secondary to a previously undiagnosed arteriovenous malformation (AVM). What is the systolic blood pressure goal for this patient during transport?

a. 120 systolic
b. 130 systolic
c. 140 systolic
d. 160 systolic

Chapter 11 | Toxicology – Poisons & Toxic Ingestions

1) You are transporting a 5-year-old pediatric patient who consumed a significant amount of Elavil (amitriptyline). Upon your assessment, you would expect to find what patient presentation?

   a. Bradycardia and hypotension
   b. Hyperventilation and hyporeflexia
   c. Fever and agitation
   d. Severe bradycardia and salivation

2) You arrive on scene to find a 12-year-old who overdosed on nevibolol (Bystolic) as a suicide attempt. On the monitor, you notice this:

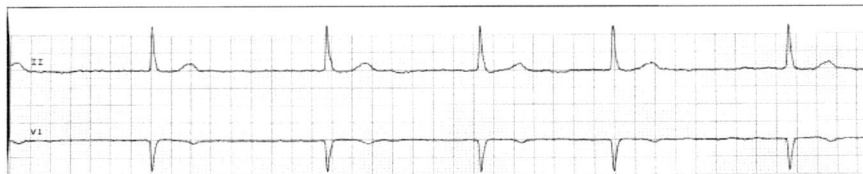

Which of the following therapies would be anticipated to be unsuccessful?

   a. Dopamine
   b. Transcutaneous pacing
   c. Atropine
   d. Glucagon

3) You are transporting a 16-year-old who ingested an unknown substance. On assessment, the patient is unconscious and you obtain the following EKG:

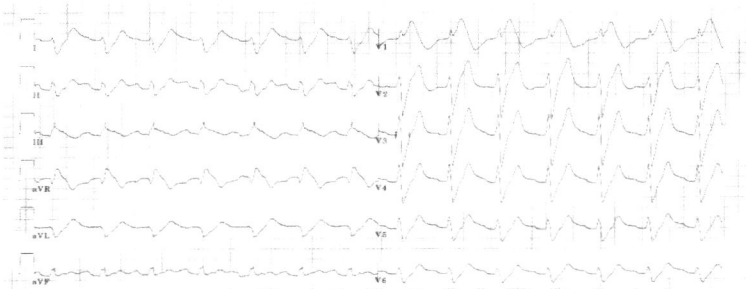

You suspect an OD related to what substance:

   a. Paxil (paroxetine)
   b. Pamelor (nortriptyline)
   c. Tenormin (atenolol)
   d. Digoxin (digitalis)

4) You arrive at a facility to transport a 16-year-old who says they took an entire bottle of acetaminophen (Tylenol). They are currently complaining of RUQ pain. Based on this presentation, when did this patient most likely ingest this drug:

   a. Less than one hour ago
   b. Within the last 1-4 hours
   c. Within the last 6-12 hours
   d. Within the last 24-72 hours

5) You arrive at a facility to transport a 14-year-old who says they took an entire bottle of an unknown drug. The patient is experiencing hallucinations. Which drug do you suspect?

   a. Benadryl
   b. Tylenol
   c. Advil
   d. Codeine

6) You have a patient who received an unintentional overdose of potassium after a medication error occurred. Their current K^+ is 7.84, pH is 7.35 and current ECG shows:

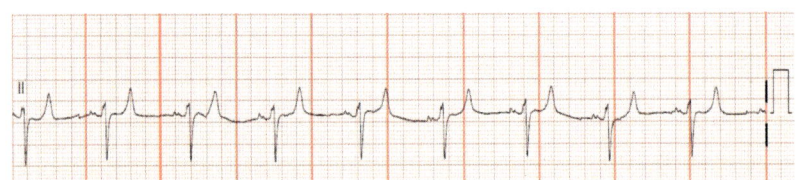

How would you manage this patient? What medications would you anticipate providing?

   1.
   2.
   3.
   4.
   5.

7) Your patient was exposed to cyanide. What antidote management would best suit this patient?

a. Physostigmine
b. Oxygen
c. Atropine and 2-PAM
d. Amyl nitrate and sodium thiosulfate

8) In an aspirin overdose, the primary acid-base disturbance would be _____ followed by _____?

a. Respiratory alkalosis; metabolic acidosis
b. Respiratory acidosis; metabolic acidosis
c. Respiratory alkalosis; metabolic alkalosis
d. Respiratory acidosis; metabolic alkalosis

9) Which medication could potentially mask early symptoms of hypoglycemia?

a. Valium
b. Verapamil
c. Metoprolol
d. Lisinopril

10) A 7-year-old patient is being transferred to a higher-level ICU. Upon obtaining an EKG, you note a prolonged QT segment. Which electrolyte would least likely be the cause of the prolonged QT?

a. Magnesium
b. Calcium
c. Potassium
d. Sodium

11) You are transporting a patient who overdosed on their prescription medication. Within minutes of your transport, you notice torsades de pointes on the cardiac monitor. Based upon this rhythm disturbance, what medication do you suspect the patient ingested?

a. Fluoxetine (Prozac)
b. Metoprolol (Lopressor)
c. Hydrocodone (Lortab)
d. Amitriptyline (Elavil)

12) A 13-year-old boy scout is brought into the ED after suffering from a snakebite to their right ankle. Time since bite is now 45 minutes. What is the most appropriate initial intervention?

a. Identify the type of snake

b. Elevate and immobilize the affected leg
c. Immobilize the extremity below the level of the heart
d. Apply ice to the skin over the snakebite wound

13) Mephedrone, Methylenedioxypyrovalerone (MDPV) and other drugs known as "bath salts" are chemically similar to:

    a. Amphetamines
    b. Benzodiazepines
    c. Barbiturates
    d. Catecholamines

14) You are called to transfer a neonate that is positive for herpes. Your first action, once you make patient contact is?

    a. Place in isolation
    b. Isolate until acyclovir is given
    c. Gloves, gown and eye protection
    d. Isolate and use standard universal precautions

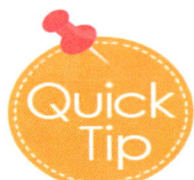

Resuscitation of your neonate and pediatric patient can be guided by the following acronym.

S – Sugar
T – Temperature
A – Airway
B – Blood pressure
L – Lab values
E – Emotional support

Karlson, K. *S.T.A.B.L.E program (6th Ed)*

Chapter 12 | Neonatal Defects, Hick-ups – Surgical Emergencies

1) You are transporting an 8-month-old infant with a 3-day history of vomiting and mucous, jelly-like stool. The infant has intermittent intense distress. On exam you note a sausage shaped mass in the RUQ. Your initial differential diagnosis is?

    a. Acute appendicitis
    b. Toxic mega colon
    c. Fecal impaction
    d. Intussusception

2) You are transporting an 8-month-old infant with a history of projectile vomiting. On exam you note sunken fontanels, dry mucosa and poor skin turgor. You can palpate an olive shaped mass in the RUQ and notice ripples of contractions across the abdomen. Your initial differential diagnosis is?

    a. Pyloric stenosis
    b. Intussusception
    c. Fulminant pancreatitis
    d. Splenic engorgement

3) Your team is assisting in the resuscitation of a 32-week-old neonate. Maternal history is unremarkable with notable exception of polyhydramnios. After an attempt at feeding, the neonate is distressed, choking, with drooling noted and secondary cyanosis. You attempt to clear the airway and place a nasogastric (NG) tube. However, the NG tube cannot be passed. What is your suspected diagnosis?

    a. Meconium aspiration
    b. Neonatal laryngospasm
    c. Tracheoesophageal fistula
    d. Bronchospasm

4) You are transporting a neonate suffering from choanal atresia. You know that your patient will have difficulty with all of the following EXCEPT?

    a. Sleeping
    b. Breathing
    c. Feeding
    d. Diuresis

5) Your patient is reported to have transposition of the great vessels. It is essential to the survival of the neonate to maintain?

   a. Oxygen
   b. PDA patency
   c. Indomethacin
   d. Oxytocin

6) The equation for determining ETT size in a pediatric patient >1-year-old is?

   a. (12 + 4) / 4
   b. 16 + 2) / 2
   c. (16 + age) / 4
   d. (16 + age) (4)

7) When giving a neonate prostaglandin (PGE1), a potential complication to administration is?

   a. Closure of the PDA
   b. Apnea
   c. Pulmonary HTN
   d. Metabolic acidosis

8) Pediatric patients will not demonstrate hypotension secondary to hemorrhage, until approximately _____ loss of blood volume.

   a. 5%
   b. 15%
   c. 25%
   d. 35%

9) Your 4kg neonate starts presenting with a repetitive mouth and tongue movement, bicycling motion, eye deviation and rapid blinking. What type of seizure would this represent?

   a. Clonic
   b. Tonic
   c. Myoclonic
   d. Subtle

10) The high vascular resistance in the fetal lung is due to the following physiologic mechanisms?

   a. Changes in O_2 tension
   b. Changes in pH and CO_2 tension
   c. Pulmonary arterial vasoconstriction
   d. Increase in systemic vascular resistance

11) During transport of a neonate, which of the following findings would indicate that the neonate is in stress?

   a. Sucking
   b. Fist clinched
   c. Hiccoughing or sneezing
   d. Quiet and alert

12) Increased irritability, increased heart rate and blood pressure, eye fluttering and decreased SpO_2 may be subtle signs of?

   a. Seizures
   b. Congenital heart defect
   c. Hydrocephalus
   d. Neurological anomaly

13) You are transporting a 32-week premature neonate with respiratory distress. Which drug may be administered in preparation for transport?

   a. Antibiotics
   b. Surfactant
   c. D10
   d. Prostaglandin

14) Your patient is PDA dependent. This would indicate that your patient would likely require the administration of which of the following drugs?

   a. Indomethacin
   b. Progesterone
   c. Prostaglandin
   d. Synthetic surfactant

15) You are called to transport a 5-day-old neonate. On arrival, your report states that the baby is suffering from Tetralogy of Fallot (TOF). You know that this congenital defect causes severe hypoxia. What is the long-term treatment to correct the heart defect?

    a. Prostaglandin (PGE1) administration
    b. High flow oxygen
    c. Catheterize and dilate the pulmonary artery (PA) and patch the Ventricular Septal Defect (VSD)
    d. Indomethacin for Patent Ductus Arteriosus (PDA) closure

16) Which of the following congenital disorders results in a right-to-left shunt?

    a. Patent Ductus Arteriosus (PDA)
    b. Isolated Ventricular Septal defect (VSD)
    c. Tetralogy of Fallot
    d. Atrial Septal Defect (ASD)

17) The primary physiologic stimulus that causes closure of the PDA is?

    a. Prostaglandin
    b. Oxygen
    c. Indomethacin
    d. Lasix

18) The most common congenital heart defect in neonates is?

    a. Patent ductus arteriosus (PDA)
    b. Aortic stenosis
    c. Tetralogy of Fallot
    d. Ventricular septal defect (VSD)

19) What is the appropriate un-cuffed ETT size for a 4-year-old-patient?

    a. 4.5 ETT
    b. 4.0 ETT
    c. 5.0 ETT
    d. 5.5 ETT

20) What is the appropriate ETT depth of insertion for a 5.0 ETT?

   a. 10 cm
   b. 11 cm
   c. 15 cm
   d. 18 cm

21) A 2-week-old infant present with lethargy, abdominal tenderness and bilious vomiting. No masses are observed or palpated on exam. You suspect?

   a. Intussusception
   b. Gastrochisis
   c. Pyloric stenosis
   d. Midgut volvulus

22) You are called to a 1.2kg neonate that was delivered at 28-weeks. The neonate presents with lethargy, abdominal distention, positive guaiac test and free air in the small and large bowel on x-ray. Labs show leukopenia, thrombocytopenia and metabolic acidosis. What is your initial differential diagnosis?

   a. Gangrenous gastrochisis
   b. Volvulus neonatorum
   c. Necrotizing enterocolitis
   d. Septic omphalocele

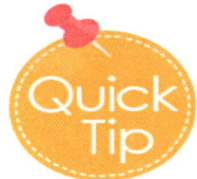

Once resuscitation has started, use THE-MISFITS acronym in an attempt to identify underlying causes.

T – Trauma, thermal, tumor
H – Hypoxia, heart disease, hypotension
E – Electrolyte disturbances

M – Metabolic derangements
I – Inborn errors of metabolism
S – Sepsis
F – Formula mishaps
I – Intestinal catastrophes
T – Toxins
S - Seizures

Retrieved from: http://pemplaybook.org/podcast/the-undifferentiated-sick-infant/

23) Your team is resuscitating a 2-day-old, 34 post-conceptual age neonate that has abdominal swelling, vomiting and has not passed meconium via bowel movement. X-ray is below. What is your suspected diagnosis?

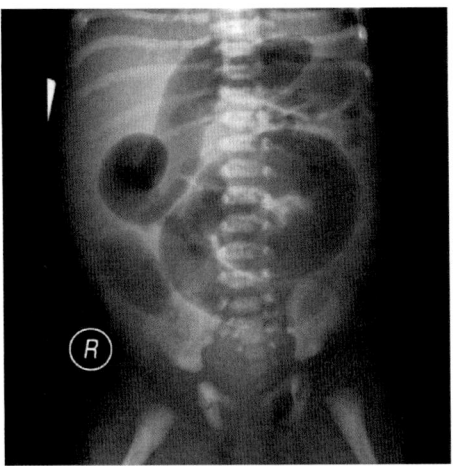

https://radiopaedia.org/cases/hirschsprung-disease-1

   a. Volvulus neonatorum
   b. Septic omphalocele
   c. Necrotizing enterocolitis
   d. Hirschsprung

24) You are resuscitating a neonate with an omphalocele. You note increased respiratory rate, mottled skin and a weak cry. What is the likely cause of this deterioration?

   a. Gastric distention
   b. Pain
   c. Hypothermia
   d. Sepsis

25) What would be the best position for a neonate with a myelomeningocele?

   a. Flexion
   b. Extension
   c. Neutral
   d. Prone

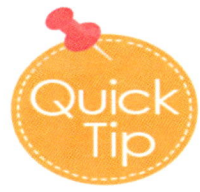

Understanding the different neonatal heart defects and their underlying pathophysiology can be overwhelming. They all share a common theme and have ductal lesions along with other manifestations. However, maintaining a patent ductus is essential. It is the only way your neonate will remain oxygenated and have a reduction in pressure based on left-sided outflow obstructions. Oxygen is the main way our body responds to close the ductus. Due to this, maintaining the lowest possible FiO_2 is important. It is not abnormal to have SpO_2 readings in the 70% range throughout the care of the neonate. Prostaglandin is also administered to maintain patency.

Chapter 13 | Lab Values Dissected

Test	Reference Range	Function and Interpretation
Hematology		

Erythrocyte (Red Blood Cell [RBC]) count (millions of cells/mm³ [microliters])	1-3d 4-6.6
	1wk 3.9-6.3
	2wks 3-5.4
	1mo 2.7-4.9
	3-6mo 3.1-4.5
	6m-2y 3.7-5.3
	2-6yr 3.9-5.3
	6-12yr 4-5.2
	12-18yr
	  M 4.5-5.3
	  F 4.1-5.1
	18+yr
	  M 4.5-5.9
	  F 4-5.2
		Function: Measures the actual number of red blood cells in the blood.
		
		Increases: Increased RBC production, renal disease, altitude, tumors, pulmonary disease, cardiovascular disease, relative increase can occur with dehydration.
		
		Decreases: Anemia, increased cell destruction, decreased production, overhydration, bone marrow problems, malnutrition, deficiencies of iron, copper, folate and/or vitamin B.

Hemoglobin (Hgb) (g/dL)	1-3d 14.5-22.5
	2m-6y 9-14
	6-12yr 11.5-15.5
	12-18yr
	  M 13-16
	  F 12-16
	18+yr
	  M 13.5-17.5
	  F 12-16
		Function: Measures the total amount of oxygen-carrying proteins in the blood.
		
		Increases: Similar to those listed under erythrocyte count. Levels >20g/dL can cause hemoconcentration and thrombosis.
		
		Decreases: Similar to those listed under erythrocyte count, anemia, hyperthyroidism, cirrhosis, severe hemorrhage, systemic diseases. Levels < 5g/dL can lead to heart failure.

			Function: Measures the percentage of an individual's total blood volume consisting of erythrocytes.

Hematocrit (Hct) (% packed erythrocyte volume [erythrocyte volume/whole blood x100])	1d
	2d
	3d
	2m-6y
	6-12yr
	12-18yr
	  M
	  F
	18+yr
	  M
	  F
		48-69
		48-75
		44-72
		28-42
		35-45
		
		37-49
		36-46
		
		41-53
		36-46
			Increases: Similar to those listed under erythrocyte count, erythrocytosis, severe dehydration, shock. Levels >60% can cause problems with thrombosis.
			
			Decreases: Similar to those listed under erythrocyte count, blood loss. Levels < 15% can cause cardiac failure.

Leukocyte (White Blood Cell [WBC]) Count (x1000 cells/mm^3 [microliter]) **Consists of 5 types:**	Birth 24hr 1mo 1-3yr 4-7yr 8-13yr Adult	9-30 9.4-34 5-19.5 6-17.5 5.5-15.5 4.5-13.5 4.5-11	Function: Measures the number of WBCs in the blood. Essential for defense against infections and plays a role in allergies and inflammation. Increases: Response to underlying disease, leukemia, corticosteroid treatment, strenuous exercise, tissue damage (burns), inflammatory disease states, severe stress. Decreases: Overwhelming bacterial infection (sepsis), bone marrow deficiency, liver or spleen disease, immunosuppressive agents, viral infections.
~ Neutrophils (%)	"Bands" "Segs"	3-5 54-62	Function: Defend against bacterial or fungal infections. Most commonly seen in the early stages of acute inflammation as well. Bands are immature while segmented are more mature

			forms. Increases: Bacterial infections. Decreases: Viral infections.
~ **Eosinophils** (%)	All ages	1-3	Function: Defend against parasitic infections and allergic reactions. Increases: Allergic responses and parasitic infections.
~ **Basophils** (%)	All ages	0-0.75	Function: Defends in allergic and antigen responses by releasing histamines causing vasodilation. Increases: Allergic reactions and hematologic disorders.
~ **Monocytes** (%)	All ages	3-7	Function: Ability to phagocytose pathogens. Eventually leaves the bloodstream to become tissue macrophages. Increases: Severe and recovery stages of infections.
~ **Lymphocytes** (%)	All ages	25-33	Function: Includes B-cells, CD+4 helper T-cells, and CD+8 cytotoxic T-cells. They operate primarily in the lymphatic system. Increases: Viral infections.
Platelets (Plt) ($x10^3/mm^3$)	Newborn 1wk-adult	84-478 150-400	Function: Measures the number of platelets in the blood. Essential for normal blood clotting. Formed in the bone marrow and lives approximately 9-12 days. Increases: Malignancies, splenectomy, some anemias, collagen diseases, polycythemia vera.

		Decreases: Anemia, some infections, bone marrow lesions, CHF, chemotherapy agents, hypersplenism, massive PRBC transfusions, ITP, TTP, HIT.
	**Blood Chemistry**	
Sodium (Na$^+$) (mEq/L)	NB 133-146 Infant 139-146 Child 138-145 Adol/Adult 136-145	Function: Main electrolyte in the extracellular fluid. Helps maintain fluid balance and assists in the regulation of the acid-base balance. Increases: Increase in sodium or excessive loss of water; volume depletion (burns, diaphoresis, diuretics), GI loss (vomiting, diarrhea), osmotic diuresis (DKA, HHNK, mannitol use), DI, fever, hyperventilation/mechanical ventilation. Decreases: Sodium loss or water excess; volume depletion (burns, diaphoresis, diuretics), SIADH, volume overload (CHF, cirrhosis, kidney injury), prolonged D5W and/or ½NS use.
Potassium (K$^+$) (mEq/L)	NB 3.7-5.9 Infant 4.1-5.3 Child 3.4-4.7 Adol/Adult 3.5-5.1	Function: Major cation intracellularly. Regulated mainly by the kidneys. Essential for cardiac and CNS function by regulating muscle and nerve excitability. Increases: Decreased excretion (renal failure, potassium-sparing diuretics), increased uptake, shifts to extracellular spaces (rhabdo, hemolysis, burns), transmembrane shifts (acidosis, ACE-I, ARB, Succinylcholine, digoxin

			toxicity). Decreases: Transcellular shifts (beta agonists, theophylline, insulin), GI loss (vomiting, diarrhea, laxative use), renal loss, reduced uptake.
Glucose (Glu) **(mg/dL)**	Cord blood 45-96 Premature 20-60 Neonate 30-60 NB 40-60 1d 50-80 >1 day 60-100 Child/Adult 74-106		Function: Primary energy source for the body's cells and only energy source for the brain and nervous system. Increases: Diabetes mellitus, pancreatic disorders, endocrine disorders, drugs, acromegaly, acute stress, chronic kidney disease, hyperthyroidism. Decreases: May indicate a physiologic response or disorder in glucose metabolism, adrenal insufficiency, excessive alcohol consumption, severe liver disease, hypothyroidism, severe infections, severe heart failure, chronic kidney failure, insulin or glucose-lowering products overdose, insulin secreting tumors, starvation.
Chloride (Cl⁻) **(mEq/L)**	Cord blood 96-104 0-30d 98-113 >30d 98-107		Function: Chief anion of extracellular fluid. Necessary for potassium retention and transport of CO_2. Assists in the formation of hydrochloric acid in the GI tract. Increases: Metabolic

		acidosis, renal failure, head injury, dehydration, hyperventilation, eclampsia, anemia, cardiac decompensation. Decreases: Diuresis, GI losses (excessive gastric suctioning, vomiting, diarrhea), chronic renal failure, CHF, edema, DKA, fever.
Calcium (Ca^{++}) **(mg/dL)**	All ages 8.5-10.5	Function: Essential for blood coagulation, muscular contraction and nerve excitability. Essential for the development of bone tissue. Has a reciprocal relationship with phosphorus. Increases: Renal impairment, low phosphorus. Decreases: Diarrhea, renal failure, high phosphorus, alkalosis.
Magnesium (Mg^{++}) **(mg/dL)**	All ages 1.5-2.5	Function: Affects cardiac and neuromuscular function. Maintains electrical potential of cell membranes. Deficits normally seen with deficits in calcium and/or potassium. Increases: Dehydration, hyperparathyroidism, hypothyroidism, adrenal gland diseases, kidney failure, magnesium infusion or medications containing magnesium (antacids, laxatives). Decreases: Alcohol use, DKA, hypercalcemia, pancreatitis, kidney disease,

		hypoparathyroidism.
Phosphorus (P⁺)	NB 5.0-7.8 1yr 3.8-6.2 10yr 3.6-5.6 Adult 3.1-5.1	Function: Provides mineral strength to bone. Integral component of DNA and RNA. Plays a role in neuromuscular function and forming and storing ATP. Increases: Acidosis, hypocalcemia. Decreases: Alkalosis, diuretic use.
Blood Urea Nitrogen (BUN) **(mg/dL)**	Premature 3-25 NB 4-12 Infant/Child 5-18 Adult 6-20	Function: Measures glomerular function and production/excretion or urea. Byproduct from the breakdown of blood, muscle and protein. Increases (azotemia): Impaired renal function, CHF, salt/water depletion (dehydration), shock, infection, diabetes, MI. Decreases: Liver failure, malnutrition, excessive IVF administration, pregnancy.

Creatinine (Cr)
 	
(mg/dL)
	Cord blood 0.6-1.2
	NB 0.3-1
	Infant 0.2-0.4
	Child 0.3-0.7
	Adolescent 0.5-1
	Adult
	  M 0.7-1.3
	  F 0.6-1.1
		Function: Waste product of muscle metabolism.
		
		Increases: Impaired renal function, muscle disease, CHF, shock, dehydration, can increase temporarily as a result of muscle injury.
		
		Decreases: Can decrease slightly during pregnancy.

Serum Osmolality (mOsm/kg)	All ages 275-305	Function: Measures the amount of chemicals dissolved in the serum. Controlled partly by ADH. Increases: Dehydration, DI, hyperglycemia, hypernatremia, CVA, head trauma, uremia. Decreases: Hyponatremia, overhydration, SIADH.
Coagulation Factors		
Prothrombin Time (PT) (seconds)	Neonate 12-18 Postneonatal < 12	Function: Measurement of the time it takes for the plasma of the blood to clot. Increases: Hemorrhagic diseases of the newborn, malabsorption, lack of blood clotting factors, DIC, liver disease, warfarin use. Decreases: Increased vitamin K (supplements or high intake of foods), estrogen-containing medications.
Activated Partial Thromboplastin Time (aPTT,	Neonate 70 Postneonatal 25-40	Function: Measures the activity of the intrinsic and common pathways of coagulation.

PTT) (seconds)		Increases: Hemophilia, von Willebrand, heparin use, DIC, lack of clotting factors or autoantibodies against certain factors, severe liver disease, vitamin K deficiency, massive blood transfusion. Decreases: Improper collection (coagulation occurs within the collection tube).

Miscellaneous

Bilirubin, total (mg/dL)	Premature: Cord blood < 2 0-1d < 8 1-2d < 12 3-5d < 16 Full term: Cord blood < 2 0-1d 1.4-8.7 1-2d 3.4-11.5 3-5d 1.5-12 Adult 0.3-1.2	Function: Bilirubin occurs when the hemoglobin protein in old red blood cells gets broken down. Increases: Increased destruction of RBCs or situations involving impairment of the excretory function of the liver.
B-type Natriuretic Peptide (BNP) (pg/mL)	All ages < 100	Function: Secreted by the ventricles in response to excessive stretch. Useful to rule out acute heart failure versus COPD. Increases: Left ventricular dysfunction, arterial and pulmonary HTN, cardiac hypertrophy, valvular heart disease.
Troponin-I (ng/mL)	All ages < 0.04	Function: Present in cardiac muscle tissue and released in response to muscle damage in the heart (MI). Increases: Myocarditis, coronary anomaly, sepsis, MI, sustained tachycardia,

		pulmonary HTN, PE, CHF, strenuous exercise, chest trauma, cardiomyopathy. Usually the greater the number, the greater the damage.

FlightBridgeED, LLC

Chapter 14 | Review Question Rationale

Chapter 1 | Oxygenation, Acids & Alkalis

1) **Correct answer: C** | This would be partially compensated because the pH is not within normal range but the PaCO$_2$ is lower than normal with metabolic involvement indicating compensation is occurring. The patient is attempting to blow off the acid to protect the pH from dropping further.
2) **Correct answer: A** | This is classic uncompensated respiratory alkalosis because of the pH being high (Alk) and the PaCO$_2$ being low (not enough acid). There is no metabolic compensation. Classic first stage of shock!
3) **Correct answer: D** | For every 0.10 increase in pH, you will have a corresponding decrease in K$^+$ by 0.6. Any pediatric patient with a critically low K$^+$ should receive a dose of 0.5mEq/kg/hr for 1-2 hours, not to exceed the standard 20-40mEq/hr total dose of K$^+$ prior to trying to correct a metabolic disorder (increasing pH).
4) **Correct answer: C** | For every change in PaCO$_2$ of 10mmHg, you will have a change in pH of 0.08 in the opposite direction. This is an excellent way to correct pH in a patient with an abnormal pH.
5) **Correct answer: A** | Remember that with Bohr effect and the presence of increased acid or lower pH, your Hgb will release its load of O$_2$ to the tissues. In a right shift on the oxyhemoglobin curve, we see "R" for raised acid, temp, 2,3-DPG and PaO$_2$.
6) **Correct answer: D** | Lactate levels will increase in dehydration and muscle exertion. However, it is also the most sensitive marker for tissue perfusion and predicting mortality in sepsis and septic shock. Every point > 2.5 increases mortality by 10%.
7) **Correct answer: C** | This is a common question where you will just need to remember the formula. Always remember that any change in EtCO$_2$ will affect the pH in the opposite

direction. Formula = 10mmHg change in PaCO$_2$ will have an opposite change in pH of 0.08.

8) **Correct answer: B |** Because the pH is still in the compensatory range of 7.35-7.45, this would have a "first name" of compensated. Next, think of your last name. Anything that falls below 7.40 is an acid. So you have the first name of compensated and a last name of acidosis. Now find the middle name. Next look at the PaCO$_2$. You have a high value meaning you have too much acid. This is the respiratory component. Your HCO3⁻ is in the normal range. There is no kidney involvement. Your middle name is respiratory. This is a compensated respiratory acidosis.

9) **Correct answer: C |** Always remember that basic response we have in a stress situation. Our respiratory rate will increase and then our heart rate. This initial RR increase will cause an initial respiratory alkalosis.

10) **Correct answer: B |** This again is a recall question. Remember that an increase or decrease of HCO3⁻ of 10mEq will change the pH by 0.15 in the same direction. This response is going to have the greatest impact as it translates to correcting an abnormal pH.

11) **Correct answer: D |** Go through your steps in the ABG diagnosis. Identify the first name. This would be uncompensated because we have a pH that is outside the compensatory range of 7.35-7.45. Current pH is 7.6. Next, identify the last name. This would be an alkalosis because it is >7.45. Next, identify the middle name. Look at the PaCO$_2$. Is it normal? No! It's lower than the compensatory range of 35-45. So you know that a lower PaCO$_2$ tells you that you're losing acid. Double-check the HCO3⁻. Is it normal? No! Your kidneys are not able to excrete the HCO3⁻. Your middle name is then mixed. Your correct answer is a mixed disturbance.

12) **Correct answer: B |** Remember your rule. A 10mmHg change in PaCO$_2$ will change the pH by 0.08 in the opposite direction. You have a drop of 20mmHg in the EtCO$_2$. This translates to an increase of 0.16 in the pH. Add this to the initial pH and you have a final answer of 7.26.

13) **Correct answer: C |** Recall the rules for respiratory failure. You have both of the criteria present. $PaCO_2$ >50 and associated hypoxia with the PaO_2 < 60. This patient is going downhill and needs airway intervention and good ventilator management strategies.
14) **Correct answer: C |** Whenever a patient is suffering from metabolic acidosis, there will be a shift of K^+ out of the cell and into the blood. Remember that often this is a false high and should never be treated. Center your treatment around fixing the metabolic acidosis and trend the K^+ often to identify changes. The one presentation that would make you focus on treatment of the K^+ would be in a DKA patient. DKA patients will either result in a critically low K^+ or a normal to high K^+. Always give runs of K^+ in these patients because of the fluid resuscitation and the correction of the metabolic disorder. You will shift K^+ with treatment, so make sure you give K^+ and trend labs for desired effect.
15) **Correct answer: D |** Because of how the PRBCs are stored and how they lack the properties associated with whole blood, rapid, massive transfusion will result in depletion of 2,3-DPG and thus move the oxyhemoglobin curve to the left. Remember, a curve to the left causes an increased "affinity", causing Hgb to hold onto O_2. This will cause an excellent SaO_2 saturation, but a poor PaO_2 (tissue hypoxia).
16) **Correct answer: D |** Continued NGT suctioning will cause a severe metabolic alkalosis. Metabolic alkalosis is a primary increase in serum bicarbonate (HCO_3^-) concentration. This occurs as a consequence of a loss of H^+ from the body or a gain in HCO_3^-. In its purest form, it manifests as an alkalemia (pH >7.40). As a compensatory mechanism, metabolic alkalosis leads to alveolar hypoventilation with a rise in arterial carbon dioxide tension ($PaCO_2$), which diminishes the change in pH that would otherwise occur.
17) **Correct answer: A |** This patient is suffering from a low PaO_2 and lower than desired SpO_2. All other current ventilator settings are appropriate. By increasing the FiO_2 and PEEP you increase oxygenation the quickest. Increase FiO_2 to 1.0 and PEEP to 8 and then re-evaluate.

18) **Correct answer: B |** SpO_2 is reflective of how much O_2 is attached to the Hgb. SaO_2 refers to how many Hgb are saturated.
19) **Correct answer: C |** You should have identified the first name as uncompensated, middle name as metabolic and the last name of acidosis. You also need to look at the $PaCO_2$. It's low and showing that the patient is attempting to compensate for the metabolic disorder by blowing off CO_2 using the respiratory buffer system. So you should have identified a partially compensated metabolic acidosis.
20) **Correct answer: C |** The classic identifying parameters for diagnosis of acute respiratory failure are PaO_2 < 60 and a $PaCO_2$ >50.
21) **Correct answer: D |** Think "R". Shifts to the right are caused from things raised. Remember the definition of the Bohr effect. The Bohr effect states that Hgb will unload its O_2 when there is raised acid. The Hgb will have decreased affinity. So you will have a low SpO_2 and a high PaO_2. So anything raised: raised 2,3-DPG, hyperthermia, raised CO_2, raised PaO_2 and raised acid will cause a right shift.
22) **Correct answer: C |** When we think about the left shift, allows think "L" for low or left. Decreased 2,3-DPG, hypothermia, low CO_2 and low PaO_2 will cause the Hgb to hold onto O_2. This causes a higher affinity. You will see a great SpO_2 and a poor PaO_2 leading to a false sense of oxygenation. You think the patient is oxygenating fine, when actually the patient has tissue hypoxia.
23) **Correct answer: C |** While giving patients massive transfusions secondary to hemorrhage, you need to understand that guiding overall resuscitation on blood replacement is wrong. Resuscitation should be guided on lactate and base deficit levels. While giving many units of PRBCs, the patient can become hypothermic. In addition, the citrate added to the PRBCs kill off the 2,3-DPG. This causes the Hgb to lose the ability to release oxygen to the tissues and drives the oxyhemoglobin curve to the left. This in turn causes cellular hypoxia. We think by giving PRBCs

that we are increasing oxygen carrying capacity, but we can cause other issues if not careful. The second aspect to consider would be to give prophylactic calcium replacement as well. Remember, citrate binds with calcium and magnesium and causes the patient to have decreased levels. By giving the calcium, you will increase SVR and help with contractility in the shock patient.

24) **Correct answer: D |** When understanding the oxyhemoglobin dissociation curve, the clinician knows that pH, 2,3-DPG levels, body temperature, and massive transfusions with PRBCs all play a significant role in hemoglobin's affinity, or lack of, for oxygen. Cardiac output plays no direct role in this phenomenon.

25) **Correct answer: B |** The bicarbonate buffer system is important in the acid-base homeostasis of the body. In this system, CO_2 combines with H_2O to form carbonic acid (H_2CO3). This rapidly dissociates to form hydrogen (H^+) ions and bicarbonate ($HCO3^-$).

26) **Correct answer: C |** Hydrogen ions will cause a state of acidosis. All other choices will lead to a state of alkalosis.

27) **Correct answer: D |** In the early (hyperdynamic) phase of septic shock, oxygen delivery is increased but the tissues cannot extract and use the oxygen, therefore the consumption is decreased and the venous oxygen saturation would be increased.

28) **Correct answer: A |** This formula is the standard in the critical care environment to identify how much oxygen is delivered per minute as well as how much oxygen is dissolved in the plasma. Remember that 98% of oxygen is bound to Hgb, with the remainder dissolved in the plasma. The body uses the stored oxygen in the plasma first, and then if needed, pulls oxygen from the hemoglobin. This formula is great to use in conjunction with the Fick formula to trend the SvO_2, and compare that with the amount delivered. In most sepsis patients, supply and demand are not equal, with the demand often exceeding the supply.

29) **Correct answer: C |** This patient fits the definition of "right shift". This means that the affinity between Hgb and oxygen is decreased. In the presence of high acid and/or high

concentrations of carbon dioxide, your patient will have a shift to the right. This patient's ABG reflects a partially compensated respiratory acidosis with hypoxemia. The ABG is partially compensated based on the underlying respiratory acidosis, with the associated increase seen in the HCO_3^-.

FlightBridgeED, LLC

Chapter 2 | Respiratory – Breathing & Wheezing

1) **Correct answer: C |** Decadron is a corticosteroid used to decrease inflammation. Albuterol, Terbutaline, and ketamine all have bronchodilating effects when administered.
2) **Correct answer: B |** Polycythemia can result from a small drop in HbF, that leads to a big drop in SpO_2. Polycythemia may also result if the newborn receives too much blood from the placenta at birth, as may occur if the newborn is held below the level of the placenta for a time before the umbilical cord is clamped.
3) **Correct answer: D |** A shift in the trachea away from the needle would indicate a worsening tension pneumothorax with greater tracheal deviation. All other choices are indicators of improvement after the procedure is performed.
4) **Correct answer: C |** Tingling and sensory changes are not an anticipated finding or side effect from the administration of Albuterol. All other findings are commonly seen after the medication has been administered.
5) **Correct answer: A |** Ground glass opacities can indicate many things including infection, pulmonary edema and cellular inflammation. Look at the presentation. There is no indication of pulmonary edema or CHF. This would be indicated based on a possible cyanotic outflow obstruction heart defect. Due to the prematurity, surfactant is lacking and causing alveolar collapse. This is causing hyaline membrane disease, which is very similar in pathophysiology to ARDS.
6) **Correct answer: D |** The "barking" cough, non-productive in nature, would be the initial suspicion for croup, with confirmation via chest x-ray. The steeple sign will be the diagnostic identifier on the chest x-ray and treated with racemic epinephrine in most cases.
7) **Correct answer: D |** Ketamine has bronchodilating properties and is useful in asthma patients. Using IV ketamine will result in general anesthesia without significant respiratory depression. Bronchodilation begins within

minutes of administering the medication and lasts approximately 20-30 minutes after cessation of the medication. In addition, ketamine has great analgesic effects along with sedative effects and is very good with patients that have hemodynamic instability. When administering Ketamine in the pediatric population, monitor for hypersalivation, as this is a common side effect. If you identify hypersalivation, Atropine 0.02mg/kg should be administered and suctioning performed as needed.

8) **Correct answer: C** | The treatment for respiratory acidosis should revolve around identifying the cause of hypoventilation. This acid-base disorder is secondary to higher than normal $PaCO_2$ levels.

9) **Correct answer: C** | Lactate is not a marker of tissue hypoxia like once thought. However, lactate is an indicator of stress and will increase in response to any "stress" event. In association with illness, sepsis or ARDS for example, elevated lactate signifies the body's response to the illness. The goal is to see lactate clearance and a reduction. This signifies that the body's stress response is becoming smaller.

10) **Correct answer: B** | Recall that approximately 98% of oxygen is attached to Hgb, so SaO_2 is a more accurate reading of the amount of oxygen in the blood. The PaO_2 represents only about 2% of the oxygen dissolved in the plasma. When measuring cardiac output (CO), it is a reflection of how well the heart is pumping the blood with the hemoglobin and oxygen attached. The SvO_2 is associated with the oxygen reserve and is what is left over after the tissues have extracted the oxygen they need. The MAP is a calculation reflecting organ tissue perfusion but does not have any indication regarding the amount of oxygen in the blood.

11) **Correct answer: A** | This patient is presenting with an acute respiratory obstructive process. This presentation and management is about optimizing the patient's ability to exhale. The ABGs would most often show an uncompensated respiratory acidosis, with a normal or elevated PaO_2. The patient will only become hypoxic if their

minute ventilation (V_E) becomes deficient and gas exchange is decreased.

12) **Correct answer: A** | Cyanide can be found in everyday items such as insulation, furniture coverings and carpets. These items can release cyanide if they catch fire. High temperatures and low oxygen concentrations favor the formation of cyanide gas. Cyanide impedes the aerobic metabolism process during ATP formation in the electron transport chain causing an anaerobic state.

13) **Correct answer: A** | Cyanotic heart defects, such as hypoplastic left heart are dependent on ductal flow. As such, prostaglandin administration at 0.05-0.1mcg/kg/min, given concurrently with the practice of limiting the FiO_2. Increased $FiO_2 > 0.21(21\%)$ will cause decompensation in your neonate. Increased FiO_2 administration will lead to increased pulmonary blood flow and worsening pulmonary hypertension and shunt. In these patients, gas mixing is essential in an effort to reduce the FiO_2 to a level < 0.21, with targets of 0.18-0.19 often seen.

14) **Correct answer: C** | Looking at the patient's ventilation status identifies acute respiratory failure. Any $PaCO_2$ level that is above 50mmHg is an indicator of respiratory failure. In addition, a PaO_2 of < 60mmHg is an indication of hypoxic respiratory failure.

15) **Correct answer: B** | Remember the concept of absorptive atelectasis. Nitrogen is 78% of atmospheric air. It's very dense and doesn't diffuse in low O_2 states (21%). In high concentrations however, it will be displaced by O_2. Use the rule of $5 \times FiO_2 = PO_2$!

16) **Correct answer: A** | Remember, a good way to determine tube depth after watching it go through the cords, is 3 x tube size.

17) **Correct answer: D** | In infants that are 48-weeks post conceptual age (8 weeks old) with RSV, apnea is a major risk factor and should be watched closely. Prophylactic intubation is not necessary. Just be ready and have your equipment/medications available.

18) **Correct answer: B** | RSV kids do not need Albuterol or Atrovent like once thought. Only 1 out of 4 kids will respond.

The best approach is nebulized-humidified normal saline and suctioning as needed.

Chapter 3 | Ventilation, Ventilators and "Baby Lungs"

1) **Correct answer: A** | PIP being elevated with a normal P_{plat} is a direct indication of upper airway involvement: volume, flow, airway constriction, pulmonary toilet, ETT kink, or vent circuit kink! Think above the carina!
2) **Correct answer: C** | Pressure control ventilation, although very good for hypoxic patients, or patients with poor chest compliance ("baby lungs"), is based on lung compliance, so you do not have a guaranteed minute ventilation (V_E). The tidal volume (V_t) will change based on changes with chest wall compliance.
3) **Correct answer: B** | P_{plat} is the most sensitive marker for alveolar health. Trending the P_{plat} during initial ventilator set up and throughout your care is essential to identify high pressures that will damage the lungs and alveoli and cause ventilator induced lung injury (VILI), inflammatory cascades and barotrauma.
4) **Correct answer: C** | SIMV is the most dynamic mode of ventilation and provides three levels of ventilator support. First, it will guarantee a minute ventilation (V_E) for an apneic patient. Second, it will allow the patient to take spontaneous breaths based on the trigger and augment those spontaneous breaths with the addition of pressure support (PS). Third, it will allow the patient to completely control the ventilator if the patient has the necessary respiratory drive.
5) **Correct answer: C** | Airway pressures are the most important parameter to monitor on your ventilated patient. PIP, P_{plat} and static compliance reveals many things as it relates to alveolar health, barotrauma and overall lung health.
6) **Correct answer: C** | With any metabolic acidosis, always remember to allow the patient to compensate. If the patient is paralyzed, then match their respiratory rate and $EtCO_2$ reading prior to intubation so as to continue blowing off

excess acid (CO_2). This will prevent the pH from decreasing. Remember the Winter's formula. For every 10mmHg of change in $PaCO_2$, you will have an inverse change in pH by 0.08.

7) **Correct answer: B** | When attempting to increase oxygenation in patients that are hypoxic, always increase the FiO_2 first and PEEP second. With the answers available, increasing PEEP would be your best choice.

8) **Correct answer: D** | When you look at ventilator pressures, always look first at the PIP. This looks at volume, compliance, airway resistance and flow. If this is high, then check your P_{plat}. If this reflects low, you know that this elevation in pressure is due to something above the carina. If the PIP is high and you have a P_{plat} that is high as well, remember the elevated P_{plat} is causing the transient pressure change in the upper airways, and the problem is at the alveolar level.

9) **Correct answer: C** | Dead space is an aspect that many forget to account for. If not accounted for, you will cause hypoventilation. Remember that for each breath you lose approximately 150mL per breath. Using the 1mL per pound of ideal body weight for your dead space calculation, you will allow for this and increase your minute ventilation (V_E) to account for this loss. Understanding that overall V_E is different than alveolar minute ventilation (V_A) is important when looking at what's accounting for gas exchange.

10) **Correct answer: B** | The PaO_2 is low on this patient. This problem can be improved by increasing the FiO_2 or PEEP. Because the FiO_2 is already at 0.6 and the PEEP is only at 5, an increase in the PEEP would be the most preferable choice because this is most likely ARDS. In most patients, increasing the FiO_2 would be your first choice. However, remember that increasing FiO_2 for long periods leads to the release of free radicals, causes nitrogen washout and atelectasis trauma and will worsen the inflammatory cascade already in full effect from the surgery. A PEEP of 5 is considered physiologic, not therapeutic. You should make the effort to limit the amount of FiO_2 that the patient requires to the least amount possible to prevent oxygen toxicity over a period of time.

11) **Correct answer: A** | This would be a mixed disturbance because you have respiratory and kidney involvement showing acidosis. Your $PaCO_2$ is 70 and HCO_3^- 14.

12) **Correct answer: C** | Pressure regulated volume control uses volume targeted-pressure limited delivery to achieve V_t. The ventilator is constantly checking compliance and volume to regulate the pressure to achieve the desired V_t. This is very safe, effective and gentle for patients.

13) **Correct answer: D** | When treating a patient with any obstructive lung disease, remember that the number one objective is to allow the patient optimal time to exhale. In the patient presentation, using an I:E ratio of 1:4 is the best option. This approach, along with lowering the patient's (f) will allow the patient optimal time to blow off the retained $PaCO_2$.

14) **Correct answer: D** | With the sudden increase seen in peak inspiratory pressure (PIP), you should always immediately check the plateau pressure (P_{plat}). If the P_{plat} is >30 mmHg in this patient, immediate chest decompression should be your first priority. The D.O.P.E pneumonic should be utilized as well, but the increase in P_{plat} is indicating an increase in alveolar pressure and warrants correction.

15) **Correct answer: D** | Using SIMV has become the primary mode of ventilation when dealing with patients that are ventilator dependent. Research has shown that assist control causes respiratory muscle atrophy and severely hinders patients being weaned off the ventilator. SIMV is now used around the country for a primary mode because it always allows the patient the ability to take some type of spontaneous breath. With the addition of pressure support (PS), the patient is able to take an augmented breath and it reduces the work of breathing. The objective is to allow some patient induced respiratory effort, without causing muscle fatigue. It's important to establish a PS reading that is at least 5 cmH_2O greater than your current PEEP. So, if your PEEP is set at 5 cmH_2O, then set your PS at a minimum of 10 cmH_2O. This helps eliminate dead space that is currently in the ETT and ventilator circuit. You then want

to monitor those spontaneous breaths. You don't want the patient's spontaneous breaths to exceed 75% of your set V_t. So, if your V_t is set at 400 mL, your patient's spontaneous breath shouldn't exceed 300 mL. If this happens, treat the patient with an analgesic medication and sedation.
16) **Correct answer: B |** Ketamine is the only medication in the list that has beta-2 stimulation properties and optimizes bronchial dilation.
17) **Correct answer: D |** Prematurity is the key here. Surfactant replacement is needed to maintain alveolar recruitment. Air leak syndrome is common and can occur based on more the prematurity than the surfactant replacement. There is often a very rapid improvement in gas exchange in surfactant treated infants who are surfactant deficient. This is accompanied by dramatic improvements in static pulmonary compliance and lung mechanics.
18) **Correct answer: B |** This is a classic chest x-ray showing bilateral "ground glass" appearance. This is also matched with prematurity and the need for surfactant therapy. These neonates will present with respiratory decompensation 3-6 hours after delivery. It's important to treat this as sepsis until cultures are back. Broad-spectrum antibiotics that hit on both gram-negative and gram-positive bacteria will be administered.
19) **Correct answer: A |** This will also be similar in appearance when compared to hyaline membrane disease. However, this will be matched by the cardiac decompensation seen in cyanotic heart defects once the ductus closes. This normally manifests 3-5 days after birth. Pulmonary hypertension and edema will be present, along with cardiogenic shock signs and symptoms.
20) **Correct answer: C |** You'll note the appearance of bowel and air in the upper left side of the chest x-ray. Diaphragmatic hernia is a major defect and is often diagnosed in utero. This will cause secondary problems such as pulmonary hyperplasia, pulmonary hypertension and CHF.
21) **Correct answer: B |** This is classic croup, with the "steeple sign", indicating significant narrowing of the upper airway.

Croup is a viral illness and is managed with supportive care and racemic epinephrine administration.

22) **Correct answer: C** | Epiglottitis is shown in this x-ray and an easily identifiable "thumb print" sign showing an inflamed epiglottis. Epiglottitis is a bacterial infection and much more common now days in adults than children. Lower economic areas may have higher pediatric incidence because of low compliance with childhood vaccinations in comparison to middle and higher economic areas of the United States.

23) **Correct answer: C** | This pediatric patient is suffering from a right lung tension pneumothorax. You can see the high amount of black, with no visible vascular markings and deflation of the right lung into the hilar area.

Chapter 4 | Flight Physiology

1) **Correct answer: B |** In these types of questions, always take the least amount of time if it's above 35,000 ft. MSL.
2) **Correct answer: A |** Think of how your tires on your car expand in the summer and decrease in size during the winter months. As you increase the temperature, the air in an enclosed space will expand. You can also relate this to your cascade O_2 cylinder. As the temperature increases throughout the day, the amount of O_2 pressure in the tank will increase proportionally.
3) **Correct answer: A |** Dalton's law (or Dalton's gang) essentially states that as we ascend in altitude, the concentration of O_2 remains the same. However, because of the decreased barometric pressure, the partial pressure (PaO_2) of oxygen decreases as the altitude increases. So, in the simplest terms, imagine if you had a zip lock bag filled with oxygen molecules. At sea level, the oxygen molecules would have a greater pressure exerted against them (760 torr). At 18,000 ft., the same concentration of oxygen would have 380 torr of pressure exerted against the oxygen molecules, thus the partial pressure becomes very low. That same amount of oxygen at sea level would have a partial pressure (PaO_2) of 159. However, the PaO_2 would only be 79 at 18,000 ft. See example below.
   At sea level: 760 torr x 0.21 = 159 PaO_2
   18,000ft: 380 torr x 0.21 = 79 PaO_2
4) **Correct answer: C |** Giving high concentrations of O_2 is affecting Henry's law and the solubility of oxygen diffusion. Graham's law affects the active process of diffusion, which is moving from a higher concentration to a lower concentration. Henry's law is affecting the concentration, the solubility and the pressure that oxygen molecules need to be placed under to diffuse more rapidly into a solution (blood).
   Remember the rule of FiO_2 x 5 = Potential PaO_2
5) **Correct answer: D |** As we ascend in altitude the barometric pressure decreases. This allows more gas to

occupy a space. Boyle's law states that as we increase in altitude the volume increases as barometric pressure decreases. An expanding ETT is an indication of volume increasing due to the decreasing atmospheric pressure. Boyle's law is in play.

6) **Correct answer: B |** When thinking about this gas law always think about a carbonated drink. The drink, when unopened, has a higher amount of pressure above the solution. When you open the drink, the pressure above the fluid immediately equalizes with the atmosphere becoming lower than the pressure of the gas dissolved in the beverage. Additionally, we need to understand that this is our most important gas law as it relates to oxygenation. We can apply it by doing three things. First, increase the concentration. By increasing FiO_2 to 100%, you in-turn start driving up the PaO_2. Next, we need to increase the surface area by adding PEEP. If we increase the alveolar membrane's size, we then have more area for gas exchange. Last, we put the solution under pressure. By adding positive pressure via a BVM or the ventilator, we then push those increased O_2 molecules through the solution (blood).

7) **Correct answer: C |** At sea level, the dissolved gases in the blood and tissues are in proportion to the partial pressures of the gases in the person's lungs at the surface. As the diver descends underwater, the ambient pressure increases, and therefore the pressure of the gas inside the lungs increases correspondingly. Because the partial pressures of the gases in the lungs are now greater than the dissolved partial pressures of these gases in the blood and tissues, gas molecules begin to move from the lungs into the blood and tissues. Eventually, the concentration of the dissolved gases in the blood and tissues will be proportional to the partial pressures in the breathing gas (i.e., a state of equilibrium). However, if the diver resurfaces too quickly, as the pressure decreases as he/she comes to the surface, the excess nitrogen can't be dissolved in the lungs quick enough causing decompression sickness. This causes the possibility of the bends, creeps, chokes and staggers.

8) **Correct answer: C |** Charles's law states that a change in temperature will cause a change in volume. If you were to let a balloon increase in altitude, that balloon would have a decrease in volume as temperature decreases. For every 1000 feet increase in altitude, the temperature decreases by 2°C.
9) **Correct answer: A |** For every 1000 feet increase in altitude, the temperature decreases by 2°C. You may see it also referenced as: For every 150m ascended, temperature decreases 1°C. This calculates as: 150m x 3.3ft = 495ft. 495' x 2 = 990' and 2°C drop in temperature. This is the same as saying 1000' increase, 2°C drop in temperature.
10) **Correct answer: D |** Based on our increase in altitude and corresponding decrease in atmospheric pressure, Boyle's law states that the volume in the bag of saline will increase. This in turn will cause the drip rate to increase as well. It will then decrease as we descend. Based on this, you should place the bag in a pressure bag, pump it up to a moderate level and then use your dial to adjust the flow rate. Utilizing this method allows you to overcome the increases and decreases seen in altitude changes and the effects of Boyle's law. Thus, allowing your drip rate to be more consistent.
11) **Correct answer: D |** NG/OG tube placement is warranted and indicated. As you increase in altitude, any volume will expand. The increase in respiratory rate and work of breathing is most likely from the volume expansion in the abdomen that's compressing on the diagram and lungs.

FlightBridgeED, LLC

Chapter 5 | Little Tikes Heat & Cold Injuries

1) **Correct answer: C** | All of the above are important aspects of how we compensate. However, glycogen stores will limit the neonate's ability to shiver and produce heat.
2) **Correct answer: B** | With temperatures below 30°C, the medication pharmacodynamics mechanism of action will not work, thus causing the medication to build up in the system.
3) **Correct answer: Rationale** | Controlling the airway and slowing the seizure activity should be your first priority but there are several things that need to occur very early on. The seizure activity is occurring from the hyponatremia. Na^+ levels <120 mEq/L will normally be the threshold for seizure activity. Once the Na^+ is raised >120 mEq/L, most often the seizure activity will cease. Treating the hyponatremia using a 3% saline or other hypertonic fluid is going to be essential to stopping the seizure activity. However, this needs to happen very slowly in most cases. Best practice would be to raise the Na^+ enough to stop the seizure activity (usually 3-5 mEq/L) and then slowly increase it from there to get back to normal limits. Raising Na^+ levels too quickly will lead to central pontine myelinolysis. Hyponatremia should be corrected at a rate of no more than 8-10 mEq/L per day. The patient's serum osmolality is elevated secondary to a dehydrated state so initiating fluids for rehydration is essential as well which will also slowly increase the sodium (using a NS solution). Correcting the blood sugar and addressing the hypokalemia should occur as well.
4) **Correct answer: B** | Rewarming needs to take place in the most physiologic manner possible. Passive external would be removing wet cloths and using the patient's own body to warm itself via blankets. While active external would take place by a heater source, active internal rewarming would include warm humidified O_2, warm IV fluids, ECMO, gastric lavage with warm fluids and intubation.
5) **Correct answer: C** | Temperature regulation in the neonate is limited by an immature hypothalamus and poor insulating

fat called "brown fat". This is also made difficult by the large body surface area that neonates have.
6) **Correct answer: B** | All of the answers are correct except for "oxygen supply exceeds demand". In the hyperthermic patient there will be a high demand for oxygen and a low supply. We need to optimize oxygenation through all means necessary.
7) **Correct answer: C** | The earliest lab value that identifies muscle damage and release of myoglobin is going to be your CK. Creatine kinase is an enzyme that is present in all the muscles of the body and is a catalyst in the energy conversion process. Rhabdomyolysis occurs when damaged skeletal muscle releases myoglobin. Myoglobin is the oxygen carrier for the muscle tissue and is very similar to hemoglobin. However, it's very toxic when released outside of muscle tissue. Hyperthermia and prolonged seizure activity can both lead to the development.
8) **Correct answer: B** | When malignant hyperthermia manifests, it's usually in response to the administration of succinylcholine. Because of the depolarizing aspects of the medication and the fasciculations, massive calcium release can occur. This causes a sustained muscle firing throughout the body and the muscle rigidity generates excessive heat. This causes an immediate rise in body temperature.
9) **Correct answer: D** | When malignant hyperthermia manifests, it's usually in response to the administration of succinylcholine. Initial signs/symptoms will be: masseter spasms and/or trismus despite the paralytic administration, a rapidly increasing EtCO$_2$, tachycardia, and hypertension. The treatment is to administer Dantrolene sodium 2.5 mg/kg until signs/symptoms stop and begin aggressive cooling measures.
10) **Correct answer: A** | When dealing with drowning, and understanding the difference with fresh water and salt water drowning, it's important to realize that although they may seem similar, fresh water drowning causes systemic washout of the surfactant, which is important for alveolar health. Without it, atelectasis trauma and collapse will ensue. With salt water drowning, the salt causes a hyperosmolar shift and third spacing of blood and plasma

into the pulmonary spaces. This will need to be treated with your ventilator, very similar to how we treat patients with ARDS or pneumonia. Lower Vt, higher (f) and higher PEEP.

11) **Correct answer: B |** This presentation is classic for a black widow bite. Black widow venom is an ion channel poison that promotes excess release of neurotransmitters, causing the muscular and autonomic nervous system responses like hypertension and tachycardia. The key words "boardlike abdominal rigidity" should clue you into black widow!

12) **Correct answer: D |** All of the following answers are correct expect for magnesium sulfate. Black widow antivenin is made from an equine-based serum. This will always increase the possibility of anaphylaxis and serum sickness. It's important to never administer the serum until a skin test has been completed and proper consent has been established. Likewise, it is reserved for the most symptomatic cases that result in progressive respiratory decline and hypertensive crisis. Core treatment is focused on pain control, benzos, skin testing with possible antivenin administration and tetanus immunization.

13) **Correct answer: D |** The correct answer in this setting is focused on immobilizing the extremity at or below the level of the heart. This will help minimize the distribution of venom. It's not recommended to elevate the extremity above the level of the heart, as this will increase distribution. It's also not recommended to place a restricting band or ice on the bite area.

14) **Correct answer: D |** When core temperatures drop to < 30°C you would perform CPR only and start rewarming measures. Once the core temperature is >30°C you can defibrillate and provide medications if needed.

Chapter 6 | Hematology & Electrolytes

1) **Correct answer: C** | Although treatment for correction of DIC is intense and controversial, the main focus should always be treating the underlying problem. If the patient is suffering from a massive head injury, do what is necessary to correct the problem and the DIC will ultimately correct.
2) **Correct answer: C** | The H&H will normally increase by 1 & 3 with each unit of PRBCs administered. Also, remember that the Hct is approximately 3 times that of the Hgb.
3) **Correct answer: C** | Normal magnesium levels are 1.5-2.5 mEq/L. Hypermagnesemia manifestations result from depressed neuromuscular transmission. Absence of reflexes reflect a magnesium level around 7 mEq/L. Hypotension is also a manifestation.
4) **Correct answer: C** | Hypokalemia results in inverted T waves, ST segment depression, and prominent U waves.
5) **Correct answer: B** | Hypoparathyroidism causes the body to secrete low levels of parathyroid hormone. This hormone maintains and regulates calcium and phosphorus. These findings are indicative of a decrease in serum calcium. This would cause an increased phosphorus level as well, because calcium and phosphorus have an inverse relationship.
6) **Correct answer: B** | Dehydration is the most common cause of an increased hematocrit. As the volume of fluid in the blood drops, the RBCs per volume of fluid rises. The Na^+ levels also rise due to the loss of fluid or volume during a state of dehydration. Remember, it's a concentration based on the fluid.
7) **Correct answer: A** | Lasix can result in a state of hyponatremia. Signs of hyponatremia include: apprehension, abdominal cramps, diarrhea and convulsions. Oliguria and sticky mucous membranes are indicative of hypernatremia. Increases in urine specific gravity occur in states of dehydration or SIADH.
8) **Correct answer: C** | DIC occurs from over stimulation of the clotting cascade resulting in clots being formed in the body's

small blood vessels. Although these patients are at increased risk of bleeding due to the excessive clotting using up all the body's platelets and clotting factors, the primary problem is with clotting.

9) **Correct answer: B |** Citrate is used for anticoagulation in PRBCs. Rapid administration of PRBCs can lead to an accumulation of citrate. Normally, the liver metabolizes citrate quickly, but in some instances, toxicity can occur. This tends to occur in patients with liver dysfunction or neonates with immature liver function. It can result in hypocalcemia and hypomagnesemia when the citrate binds with calcium and magnesium.

10) **Correct answer: A |** In citrate toxicity, the citrate binds with calcium and magnesium and causes hypocalcemia and hypomagnesemia. These patients will present with signs of hypocalcemia, which needs to be restored. Remember, Ca^{++} is essential for vascular tone and inotropic aspects on the heart.

11) **Correct answer: C |** PRBCs are high in potassium due to hemolysis. Signs of hyperkalemia on the ECG include tall, peaked T waves and QRS complex widening.

12) **Correct answer: D |** The creatinine clearance directly reflects the GFR. It is an evaluation of the ability of the kidneys to filter waste products, such as creatinine.

13) **Correct answer: B |** DIC is a coagulopathy that will consume all platelets and clotting factors. All clotting studies are prolonged. The primary treatment for DIC is resolution of the offending agent.

14) **Correct answer: B |** If you are trying to identify the patient's metabolic disorder and you don't have an ABG to reference, the quickest calculation to identify a metabolic acidosis is via an anion gap. You can calculate an uncorrected anion gap or a corrected anion gap. See below:
Uncorrected = Na^+ - (Cl^- + $HCO3^-$) *If > 12 you have a metabolic acidosis*
Corrected = Na^+ - (Cl^- + $HCO3^-$) + K^+ *If > 20 you have a metabolic acidosis (most accurate)*

15) **Correct answer: A |** Dehydration causes an excessive loss of total body water leading to a state of hypernatremia. Hypernatremia can cause lethargy, weakness, irritability, neuromuscular excitability and edema. If left untreated, it can lead to seizures or coma.
16) **Correct answer: C |** Hypocalcemia can cause numbness and tingling in the perioral area, muscle cramps/spasms and irritability/fatigue. Two common tests for hypocalcemia include Chvostek's sign and Trousseau's sign.
17) **Correct answer: D |** All the choices expect for changes in altitude are correct triggers of sickle cell crisis. The key for these patients is to keep them hydrated, oxygenated and pain free.

Chapter 7 | Little Hearts - RPMs & PUMP

1) **Correct answer: A |** These are just simple hemodynamic parameters. Your CVP is low indicating some type of preload problem. Next look at your CI, which is also low, telling you that cardiac output is low. Next, look at the PA S/D pressures. These are also low, as well as your PCWP, telling you that left sided preload is low as well. Now you've identified that your right and left sided preload are both low with a low cardiac output. Last, look at your SVR, which is hyperdynamic. So, there is vasoconstriction in an attempt to increase cardiac output. You should be looking at simple hypovolemia. Left systolic dysfunction is wrong because you would see high PA S/D and PCWP, which you don't have. Neurogenic shock is wrong because you would see a normal cardiac index. Last, septic shock is wrong because you would see a low SVR as well as other low hemodynamic parameters. So your answer is hypovolemic shock.
2) **Correct answer: B |** Your CVP is high. This indicates higher pressures down stream or in the right ventricle. Next, your CI is low and shows a poor cardiac output. Next your PA S/D pressures are very high. This should tell you that your left heart has a problem or has backpressure. Next, your PCWP is high, telling you that your left atrial pressures are high. Remember, your PCWP is an indication of left sided preload. Last, your SVR is very hyperdynamic at 2052. This should tell you that the patient is attempting to constrict in order to increase cardiac output and overall stroke volume. This all should lead you to look at left systolic dysfunction as your diagnosis.
3) **Correct answer: C |** Your preload is low as indicated by the low CVP. Next, look at your cardiac output, which is indicated by a normal CI. Next, identify your PA S/D pressures. This tells you left ventricular end diastolic pressures. A pressure of 30/14 is a little high but not horribly high. Next, your PCWP is only 6, telling you that left

sided preload is low. Last, your SVR is low as well, so there is no compensation happening. This should look similar to the first question. You should identify a diagnosis of neurogenic shock.

4) **Correct answer: D |** Your preload is low as indicated by the CVP of only 1. Next, look at your cardiac output that's indicated by a low CI of 1.6. Next, your PA S/D is low as well. Remember, your PA is looking at your left end diastolic pressures. This shows that your left ventricle is not able to sufficiently provide enough stroke volume. In addition, your PCWP is low as well and matches your low PA pressures. Last, your SVR is only 300. There is no constriction and no compensation. I'll give you a hint. Sepsis or septic shock is the only thing that will show you low hemodynamic numbers in all categories. Your diagnosis is septic shock.

5) **Correct answer: A |** Augmentation of the left ventricle revolves around allowing the ventricle to fill properly. Often, treatment of HTN with ACE-Inhibitors and beta blockers, are first line treatments, along with digoxin for inotropic augmentation and contractility.

6) **Correct answer: D |** PCWP is a direct marker of left atrial pressure and also indirect marker of left ventricular end diastolic pressure. It's measured by wedging the PA catheter in the pulmonary artery. Always think of it as reflective of left sided preload status.

7) **Correct answer: D |** You are wedging the PA catheter to get a measurement of the left atrial pressure. When you see a V on the waveform while performing the wedge, it shows left atrial filling against a closed mitral valve and thus shows mitral valve disease/regurgitation.

8) **Correct answer: B |** When assessing your A-line, you are looking for the dicrotic notch. This is indicative of pulmonic valve closure while using the swan, and aortic valve closure while using the A-line during IABP therapy. The A-line will be used for secondary timing on your balloon pump (IABP).

9) **Correct answer: B |** Don't forget that CVP and RAP are looking at the same things. They both reflect preload. Most often the question will just use CVP. You can always identify volume status by looking at the CVP and titrating

your treatment based on those numbers. Standard CVP/RAP readings will be 2-6mmHg.

10) **Correct answer: B |** Anytime you see a low CVP always think preload issues. You can also see the cardiac index is low with an associated high SVR which should make you think volume.

11) **Correct answer: C |** When you see hemodynamic parameters that are high across the board with a low CI, that should lead you to think cardiogenic shock. These will be classified as cyanotic heart defects such as, coarctation of the aorta, hypoplastic left heart, Tetralogy of Fallot and transposition of the great vessels

12) **Correct answer: C |** Normal SVR is 800-1200 dyne-sec/cm^{-5}. This measurement is a recall type question. SVR is measured by the following formula:

$$\frac{80 * (MAP-CVP)}{Q}$$

13) **Correct answer: A |** Stroke Volume (SV) = End Diastolic Volume – End Systolic Volume. Thus, CO= SV x HR. Remember SV is made from preload, afterload and contractility.

14) **Correct answer: B |** The formula for determining MAP is: [SBP + (2 x Diastolic) / 3]

15) **Correct answer: B |** Having a good understanding of what your CVP pressure will tell you is essential in providing good patient care. Remember, your CVP will tell you if your patient is volume depleted or volume overloaded. It's that simple. You can use the CVP to guide fluid resuscitation in your sepsis patients by maintaining a CVP of 8-12mmHg or a CVP of 12-15mmHg with patients who suffer from chronic hypertension or left ventricular hypertrophy.

16) **Correct answer: D |** The SvO_2 is the most accurate way to determine tissue oxygenation and is used in the ICU setting to trend and determine central venous tissue oxygenation. We use this to determine supply versus demand. The goal is to maintain a level >70%.

17) **Correct answer: C |** The normal range for PCWP is 8-12mmHg. PCWP is a direct reflection of left atrial diastolic pressure as well as an indirect reflection of left ventricular

end diastolic pressure and tells you the status of left sided preload as well as afterload status.
18) **Correct answer: D** | Normal PA pressures are: Systolic = 20-30mmHg. Diastolic = 10-15mmHg.
19) **Correct answer: D** | Out of all of the answers, the hemodynamic parameters of PAP 44/22 and PCWP 18 are both high and should tell you the patient is overloaded and lead you to diagnose left ventricular failure or cardiogenic shock.
20) **Correct answer: C** | Central venous pressure (CVP) monitors right atrial pressure and is a direct indication of preload. CVP will always dictate fluid needs. Normal CVP is 2-6mmHg.
21) **Correct answer: D** | Elevated PA pressures are a direct indication of afterload (left atrial and ventricular end-diastolic pressures). Mitral valve regurgitation, stenosis, and left ventricular failure are all primary aspects of afterload and left ventricular function.
22) **Correct answer: B** | The values of CVP 8, CI 1.4, and PCWP 13, are all an indication of left sided failure. The CVP is high showing that there are high pressures upstream (left side are elevated). The CI is a direct reflection of CO, which tells you the left ventricular function is poor. PCWP is a direct reflection of left ventricular end diastolic pressure and is elevated. Your diagnosis should be left sided heart failure.
23) **Correct answer: B** | Anytime you identify that your patient's PA diastolic pressure is higher than their PCWP, it's an indication of pulmonary hypertension. Pulmonary hypertension is a disease process secondary to an acute hypoxic state, COPD, ARDS or pulmonary embolus.
24) **Correct answer: C** | ACE-Inhibitors block the stimulation of the renin-angiotensin-aldosterone (RAA) system. When the RAA system is stimulated by hypo-perfusion of the kidney, it causes vasoconstriction and sodium and water retention. Stimulation of the RAA system would lead to further deterioration in a heart failure patient.

25) **Correct answer: D** | Neo-synephrine is a potent alpha stimulating medication used in open-heart recovery in the neonate population. It has potent alpha effects without causing an increase in heart rate and O_2 demand.
26) **Correct answer: C** | If your assessment reveals no femoral pulses and a lower SpO_2 on the lower extremities in comparison to the upper pre-ductal SpO_2, this indicates a left side outflow obstruction defect such as, coarctation of the aorta, hypoplastic left heart, Tetralogy of Fallot and transposition of the great vessels.
27) **Correct answer: B** | Neonates are born with right axis deviation due to the high-pressure right side while in utero. Once the neonate is born, the heart switches to a high pressure left side. Right axis deviation should not be seen in the neonate greater than 1 week in most cases. In addition, you should never see a newborn in left axis deviation. This is an immediate indication of a left sided outflow obstruction defect.
28) **Correct answer: C** | Left axis deviation should never be seen in the newborn. This indicates left ventricular hypertrophy and a left sided outflow obstruction defect. Remember, neonates have a high-pressure right side in utero. When they're born they should always show right axis deviation because of this. This changes and goes to normal axis within the first week of life.
29) **Correct answer: B** | The normal starting dose for prostaglandin administration is 0.05-0.1mcg/kg/min
30) **Correct answer: D** | DiGeorge Syndrome is the key to this answer. DiGeorge is a primary immunodeficiency disease caused by T-cell deficiency, congenital heart defect and hypocalcemia.
31) **Correct answer: C** | Dopamine's alpha effects will cause coronary vasoconstriction and primary chronotropic effects. This leads to a reduction in cardiac output at doses >10mcg/kg/min.
32) **Correct answer: C** | Nitroprusside is the only medication in the list that reduces both preload and afterload. All other medications are vasopressors and will increase pulmonary vascular resistance.

Chapter 8 | Endocrine Renal – Hormones & Pee

1) **Correct answer: A |** This is a classic sign that the glucose has been dropped too quickly and cerebral edema has manifested.
2) **Correct answer: D |** With patients in DKA, it is essential to allow the patient to continue to compensate. Remember the rule, for every 10mmHg increase in $PaCO_2$, you will have a decrease in pH by 0.08. If we were to paralyze them and take away their compensatory mechanism, their $PaCO_2$ would significantly increase thus dropping the pH to levels of nonviable life. Proper ventilator strategies in this situation would be to place them on SIMV and give moderate sedation to allow the patient the ability to continue their compensatory drive. Option C would not be as beneficial due to AC and higher Vt.
3) **Correct answer: B |** Glucose should not be dropped more than 100 mg/dL per hour or 50 mg/dL in 30 minutes.
4) **Correct answer: A |** There is failure "before" the kidneys due to the hypovolemia. The kidneys are not being perfused enough, therefore are not diuresing.
5) **Correct answer: C |** A decrease in deep tendon reflexes (DTRs) indicates a drop in the pH and worsening metabolic acidosis leading to DKA. A urine pH less than 6 indicates that the kidneys are excreting acid. An increase in the HCO_3^- indicates improvement in the current acidotic state and potassium levels are expected to decrease as acidosis is corrected and potassium is shifted back into the intracellular space. This decrease to 5.2 mEq/L is still slightly above normal limits, thus would not be concerning.
6) **Correct answer: C |** Remember diabetes insipidus (DI) is caused by inadequate or no ADH production or release from the pituitary gland. This can be caused from a head injury, the use of phenytoin (Dilantin) or several other causes. The other choices are for DKA.
7) **Correct answer: D |** Once glucose levels reach 250-300 mg/dL a maintenance infusion with a dextrose containing

solution should be initiated so the glucose doesn't drop too quickly and cerebral edema is avoided.

8) **Correct answer: B |** Normal saline (0.9%) is the best initial fluid for resuscitation of dehydration and hyperglycemia. LR is incorrect because the presence of lactate is not desirable in someone with profound acidosis. ½ normal saline (0.45%) is hypotonic and will provide less BP support and will not correct dehydration as it causes an intracellular shift. Hypertonic saline (3%) creates an osmotic shift from intracellular into the intravascular space, making cellular dehydration worse.

9) **Correct answer: B |** Syndrome of inappropriate anti-diuretic hormone (SIADH) is the overproduction or release of ADH which results in increased serum retention with secondary water retention due to the stimulation of aldosterone receptors in the nephrons. This results in a dilutional hyponatremic state.

10) **Correct answer: C |** Neonates are at an increased risk for sepsis secondary to Group B strep. Expectant mothers should be tested or prophylactically treated with antibiotics if unknown Group B strep status or if testing and/or treatment hasn't been completed prior to delivery.

11) **Correct answer: D |** Diabetes insipidus occurs from a low level of ADH, so the patient loses large amounts of water. This causes an increase in serum Na^+, an increase in serum osmolality and an increase in urinary output with a decrease in urinary osmolality resulting from a decrease in urinary concentration.

12) **Correct answer: A |** These patients are dehydrated and really need the fluids. Part of the management with both of these conditions is replenishing the fluids along with managing the hyperglycemia.

13) **Correct answer: C |** Respiratory failure is common, usually in the first 72 hours, followed by hepatic failure and then renal failure.

14) **Correct answer: B |** Hyperglycemia is due to the insulin deficiency found in type I diabetics. The elevated blood sugar levels lead to a hypertonic diuresis, state of

dehydration, and elevation in the serum osmolality. There is an increase in the breakdown of fats and proteins for energy, which leads to an increase in ketones in the blood, leading to a state of ketoacidosis. The acidotic environment causes a shift of potassium to move out of the cell and into the serum causing hyperkalemia initially. As diuresis continues, the K^+ will be excreted eventually leading to hypokalemia, which is a more ominous finding.

15) **Correct answer: B |** With diabetes insipidus (DI), the classic symptoms are increased urination with a low specific gravity. The patient has normal serum glucose, so diabetes development would not be appropriate. With syndrome of inappropriate anti-diuretic hormone (SIADH), the patient's urinary output would be decreased and the specific gravity of the urine would be increased.

16) **Correct answer: C |** Diabetes insipidus (DI) occurs after there is a decrease in the amount of ADH that is being secreted. This leads to a state of polyuria because the body has no ADH to tell it to reabsorb water and sodium. With polyuria, the body gets rid of water but not as much sodium so it results in a state of hypernatremia. Also, the serum osmolality is increased because there are more electrolytes in the serum than water to balance it out. The specific gravity of the urine is decreased because the urine contains more free water than electrolytes (diluted).

17) **Correct answer: A |** Infection is the most common cause of DKA in insulin dependent patients due to the increased need for insulin during these periods. Remember, in patients with an increased oxygen demand, the liver is secreting enormous amounts of glycogen for the process of ATP production. Due to the insufficiency of insulin already in this patient, they require more insulin than normal to keep up with the production of increased glucose.

18) **Correct answer: B |** Cullen's sign consists of superficial edema and bruising around the umbilicus. It can occur with acute pancreatitis, bleeding from blunt trauma, bleeding from a ruptured abdominal aortic aneurysm, or bleeding from a ruptured ectopic pregnancy.

19) **Correct answer: C |** Ativan is the drug of choice and first line therapy in treating seizure activity in the pediatric

population. It has less respiratory depression effects and a longer half-life in comparison to Valium and Versed. Versed can cause myoclonic seizure activity in the low birth weight neonate as well.

20) **Correct answer: C |** In a patient suffering from DKA, there is an absolute insulin deficiency that causes glycogenolysis and gluconeogenesis. The gluconeogenesis causes the incomplete breakdown of free fatty acids, which result in ketones in the blood and urine. In HHNK, there is a relative insulin deficiency that causes glycogenolysis but does not cause gluconeogenesis. Therefore, tests for ketones are positive in the DKA patient and negative in the HHNK patient respectively.

Chapter 9 | Trauma – Trips, Spills, Breaks & Catastrophes

1) **Correct answer: C |** This is a classic advanced certification exam question for cardiac tamponade. In real life context, the jugular venous distention (JVD) and narrowing pulse pressure are going to be your ticket to diagnosis. None of us are good at listening to heart tones and in flight that would be difficult.
2) **Correct answer: B |** The Consensus formula is the new standard in burn fluid resuscitation management. The Consensus formula is often written in a range of 2-4mL/kg. However, pediatrics is 3mL/kg based on the dose range.
3) **Correct answer: A |** Urine output is essential in any patient. A patient that is producing urine is a patient that is perfusing. Urine output should be aimed at 0.5-1 mL/kg/hr. In patients with a risk of rhabdomyolysis, urine output should be aimed at >2 mL/kg/hr.
4) **Correct answer: C |** Rule of 9s state that the head accounts for 18% with the face and head combined, each arm is 9% totaling 18% as each arm was burned. Total BSA is 36%.
5) **Correct answer: A |** The Consensus formula states:
   kg x TBSA x 3 mL = volume/24 hours.
   Administer half of the total fluids during the first eight hours post-burn. The patient has received 300mL LR during the first 2 hours. Subtracting that from the total of 1350mL needed in the first 8 hours and taking into consideration the injury is 2 hours old, your answer is 1,050mL, at 175 mL/hr over the remaining 6 hours.
6) **Correct answer: D |** All of the above answers are correct except for vasopressin. All correct answers are used to increase urine output and to flush the kidneys. Vasopressin would do just the opposite and cause water retention.
7) **Correct answer: D |** The pelvis has multiple vessels that can become lacerated. Massive hemorrhage can lead to large volume loss in a matter of minutes. Vertical shear

pelvic fractures will cause the most significant potential vascular injuries.

8) **Correct answer: C |** The Consensus formula states:
   kg x TBSA x 3mL = volume/24 hours
   20kg x 45 x 3 = 2,700mL in the first 24 hours
   Remember that half that amount will be infused in the first eight hours after the burn.

9) **Correct answer: B |** With any burn patient, remember you can have significant K^+ shifts. With any transfer with burns >12 hours, be ready to treat any hyperkalemia that results in ECG changes.

10) **Correct answer: B |** The most appropriate treatment would be to give pain management and do a secondary assessment prior to transfer. It may be appropriate after a thorough secondary assessment to straighten the fractured extremity and re-splint in the position of function.

11) **Correct answer: C |** Acceleration-deceleration injuries cause a shearing tear of the aortic arch. Approximately 80% of patients that die within minutes of the accident have this type of large vessel tear.

12) **Correct answer: C |** Commotio cordis is caused by unexpected blunt force trauma that is non-penetrating to the left lateral chest or pericardium during the vulnerable state of ventricular repolarization causing a fatal ventricular dysrhythmia and sudden cardiac death.

13) **Correct answer: B |** Entrapment of <u>extraocular</u> muscles can occur with orbital wall/floor fractures, which can result in: restricted gaze, double vision, ecchymosis, and ptosis.

14) **Correct answer: C |** Previous failed attempt in the extremity or fracture of the extremity is a contraindication to placement.

15) **Correct answer: C |** Slipped capital femoral epiphysis (SCFE) will manifest with either chronic knee pain or hip pain. Pediatric patients may be able to walk without difficulty or need crutches if presentation is bad enough. Imagine the head of the femur separating from the femur shaft. This would be comparable to ice cream sliding off of the ice cream cone.

16) **Correct answer: D |** In the hyperthermic state, the muscles start breaking down and release creatinine kinase (CK) which is normally not found in the blood. This will be a telltale indicator that significant muscle breakdown has occurred.
17) **Correct answer: C |** The infusion of unwarmed or inadequately warmed intravenous (IV) fluids and cold blood may contribute to the multiple adverse consequences associated with hypothermia. These may include: cardiac arrhythmias, hemostasis abnormalities from impaired platelet function and impaired coagulation cascade, peripheral vasoconstriction, dehydration, decreased oxygen delivery to tissues (which impairs oxidative killing of bacteria by neutrophils and reduces the deposition of collagen during wound healing), increased red cell release of potassium with metabolic acidosis, and citrate toxicity (with blood component transfusions).
18) **Correct answer: B |** If your patient has a bronchial tree tear, often times it's at the carina. If you note on your assessment that you have subcutaneous air and decreasing SpO$_2$, the proper treatment is to advance the ETT past the carina for a right main stem intubation. This will secure an airway past the bronchial tear and allow you to ventilate the right lung. Even though this causes a right to left shunt, it's better than nothing and may buy you time.
19) **Correct answer: B |** Myoglobinuria, if left untreated, will result in acute tubular necrosis and profound renal failure. The only time myoglobin is found in the bloodstream is when it is released following muscle injury. It is an abnormal finding, and can be diagnostically relevant when found in the blood. Myoglobinuria is the presence of myoglobin in the urine, usually associated with rhabdomyolysis or muscle destruction, and can be lethal if left untreated.
20) **Correct answer: A |** 1gm/dL increase in the hemoglobin (Hgb) and 3% increase in the hematocrit (Hct) is the standard ratio of increase with administration of one unit of packed red cells. Another good way to identify your H&H ratio is to multiply your Hgb x 3, which should equal your Hct.

21) **Correct answer: D** | Administration of platelets, cryoprecipitate and FFP are the first line treatments to slow the DIC process. When patients are given massive transfusions of NS and PRBCs, all of their clotting factors get washed out. On top of that, the body's response to injury is to start an inflammatory cascade in the attempt to heal. This massive inflammatory cascade leads to the formation of small blood clots inside the blood vessels throughout the body. As the small clots consume coagulation proteins and **platelets**, normal coagulation is disrupted and abnormal **bleeding** can occur from the skin, the **gastrointestinal tract**, the **respiratory tract** and surgical wounds. The small clots also disrupt normal blood flow to organs (such as the **kidneys**), which may malfunction as a result. The pathophysiology of DIC is the same regardless of the triggering event. There have been two current studies that have proven beneficial for trauma patients where massive hemorrhage and transfusion occurs. Administration of tranexamic acid (TXA), within the first hour of the traumatic event with potential hemorrhage, has resulted in a lower incidence of DIC and an overall reduction in mortality.
22) **Correct answer: C** | The classical findings on a chest x-ray will be a widened mediastinum, apical cap, and displacement of the trachea. A normal chest x-ray does not exclude transection, but will diagnose conditions such as pneumothorax or hemothorax.
23) **Correct answer: C** | The circulating blood volume for a pediatric patient is 75-80mL/kg. Remember that it takes 25% blood loss to see clinical signs of decompensation in the pediatric patient. That seems like a lot, but considering that a 6kg neonate would only have 480mL max, a 25% loss would be 120mL. That is not much!
24) **Correct answer: A** | All EMTALA transfer forms need to be signed by the transferring physician or an authorized representative of that physician based on the facilities policy for signing the transfer form.
25) **Correct answer: B** | Fractures of the 1st-3rd ribs should indicate a great amount of force. Aortic disruption along

with C1-C2 fractures and scapular fractures can be associated with this amount of force and mechanism.
26) **Correct answer: D |** Correct placement for chest tube insertion is between the 4th and 5th intercostal space (ICS) and between mid- and anterior axillary. This is an important landmark. Migration down lower into the 5th or 6th ICS can cause liver or spleen injuries and misplacement.
27) **Correct answer: C |** Anytime you see a trauma patient that has no compensatory mechanisms manifesting, think neurogenic shock. With the age of the patient, along with the hypotension and bradycardia, this is classic neurogenic shock. This is classified as a distributive shock and if you had available hemodynamic readings you would see a low CVP, low PA pressure, low PCWP, low SVR and a normal to high CO.
28) **Correct answer: D |** Beck's triad is indicative of muffled heart tones, narrowing pulse pressures and JVD. In an increased ICP patient, you would see Cushing's triad in the patient that is herniating.
29) **Correct answer: A |** When we look at mechanism and potential injury patterns associated with different types of collisions, rear impact collisions will most likely be associated with c-spine injuries from the hyperextension of the neck especially if a headrest is not present.
30) **Correct answer: C |** When identifying potential types of shock in your trauma patients, always think about hemorrhage and potential secondary problems associated with losing large amounts of blood. Hemoglobin concentrations are essential for oxygen carrying capacity and should be watched closely. The patient will become tissue hypoxic quickly and anaerobic metabolism will ensue.

Chapter 10 | Neurological Injuries

1) **Correct answer: A |** To calculate the cerebral perfusion pressure (CPP) you need to figure out what the MAP is. MAP = ([2DBP] + SBP) / 3. CPP = MAP - ICP. This patient has a MAP of 70mmHg – ICP 29 = CPP 41.
2) **Correct answer: B |** The target CPP for a pediatric patient is 60 mmHg. CPP < 50 will cause ischemic changes to the brain and ultimate infarction. The goal is to employ H3 therapy.
    1. Hypervolemic (give volume)
    2. Hyperdynamic (administer an inotrope)
    3. Hypertensive (administer Levophed)
3) **Correct answer: A |** This is a classic advanced certification exam question. Remember, epidural bleeds will have a period of initial unconsciousness followed by a period of lucidness and then go unresponsive. Often, that last phase of unresponsiveness will lead to airway difficulties, clenched teeth and increased ICP.
4) **Correct answer: B |** Cushing's triad is an ominous sign and not often seen in the early management of our patients. This is a clear indication of severe increased ICP and if left untreated leads to herniation and death.
5) **Correct answer: A |** Diffuse axonal injury (DAI) is an ominous diagnosis and is difficult to identify. CT scans will be normal in 88% of patients. Only 12% of CT scans will show injury. However, an MRI can be used for confirmation and diagnosis, with 92% of DAIs being diagnosed through this avenue. DAI is an injury that causes severe shearing of the axons of the nerve cells throughout the brain.
6) **Correct answer: B |** You first need to determine the MAP. Standard ICP = 0-15mmHg. MAP = ([2(DBP)] + SBP) / 3. CPP = MAP – ICP. In this problem, your MAP = 73.
    CPP = 73 - 25 = 48mmHg

7) **Correct answer: B |** A stellate skull fracture occurs with multiple linear fractures radiating from the site of impact.
8) **Correct answer: B |** Epidural bleeds occur when blood accumulates between the dura-mater and the skull. Epidural bleeding is rapid because it is usually from an artery. The hallmark symptom is the patient may regain consciousness and appear completely normal only to descend suddenly and rapidly into an unconscious state.
9) **Correct answer: D |** Basilar skull fractures may present with CSF rhinorrhea, otorrhea, Battle sign and "raccoon eyes". Facial palsy, nystagmus and facial numbness are secondary and can occur due to the involvement of cranial nerves V, VI, and VII respectively.
10) **Correct answer: C |** The transducer should be leveled at the point of the patient's face which corresponds to the Foramen of Monro. This is the outer canthus of the eye. As with any other invasive transducer, the major point to remember is that it must always be leveled, so pick your mark and stick with it!
11) **Correct answer: B |** Brown-Sequard syndrome results in a loss of sensation and motor function caused by a lateral hemisection of the spinal cord. This is associated with: ipsilateral paralysis below the level of the lesion, positive Babinski sign ipsilateral to the lesion, ipsilateral loss of tactile discrimination, vibratory, and position sensation below the level of the lesion, and contralateral loss of pain and temperature sensation.
12) **Correct answer: C |** In the presence of a subarachnoid hemorrhage, it is essential to maintain a systolic BP at 140mmHg. Unlike the treatment goals associated with an intracerebral hemorrhage, which says that the systolic BP needs to be 160mmHg due to the location of the bleed and the required MAP needed to perfuse that level of the brain. In contrast, subarachnoid hemorrhages have a very high probability for re-bleeding. As such, the systolic BP and associated MAP need to be lower.

FlightBridgeED, LLC

Chapter 11 | Toxicology – Poisons & Toxic Ingestions

1) **Correct answer: C |** TCAs inhibit the reabsorption of dopamine, epinephrine, and norepinephrine. They work in a manner similar to cocaine. Therefore, the erratic behavior often seen in cocaine overdoses, are frequently seen with TCA ODs as well.
2) **Correct answer: C |** Although current PALS and ACLS guidelines still recommend Atropine for early treatment, resolution of symptoms are not expected. It is still recommended to attempt to eliminate any other factors such as increased vagal tone as well.
3) **Correct answer: B |** TCA OD will present with tachycardia progressing to QRS widening with worsening toxicity. This will eventually lead to VT, VF, or torsades de pointes.
4) **Correct answer: D |** The metabolites of acetaminophen usually take 24-48 hours to accumulate within the liver. This is when RUQ pain becomes the predominant symptom that presents.
5) **Correct answer: A |** Hallunications can be seen with Benadryl overdose. Tylenol, Advil and Codeine will not cause those symptoms.
6) **Correct answer: Rationale |** Calcium chloride IV over 5-10mins. Insulin and glucose. Sodium bicarbonate, Albuterol, and Lasix. Kayexalate and magnesium sulfate as needed as well.
7) **Correct answer: D |** Cyanide binds to cytochrome c oxidase in the electron transport chain, thus inhibiting oxygen conversion to water and stopping ATP synthesis. As a result, the chain can no longer produce ATP, which quickly leads to both CNS and cardiac insults. It takes 1-15 minutes to cause death. This causes us to move from an aerobic state to an anaerobic state. Any patients that have sustained prolonged periods in house fires that are hypoxic, despite oxygenation therapy, should be suspected of having cyanide toxicity.

8) **Correct answer: A |** Aspirin is acetylsalicylic acid, which causes a respiratory stimulant effect leading to respiratory alkalosis initially. It also causes a direct metabolic acidosis due to being an acid as well.
9) **Correct answer: C |** The sympathetic nervous system is responsible for the signs and symptoms of hypoglycemia. Medications that block the sympathetic system, such as beta-blockers, could potentially prevent an individual from experiencing these symptoms. Symptoms include: tachycardia, diaphoresis and nervousness. Beta blockers, such as metoprolol, can cause patients to become severely hypoglycemic without being able to identify the symptoms early on.
10) **Correct answer: D |** Sodium affects phase zero of the action potential which is responsible for depolarization. Calcium, magnesium and potassium all work on phase 2 and 3 of the action potential, which is responsible for repolarization. Low levels of calcium, magnesium and potassium will affect phase 2 and 3 of the action potential by slowing repolarization causing prolonged QT segments.
11) **Correct answer: D |** Amitriptyline (Elavil) is a TCA, which causes QT prolongation by inhibiting sodium uptake and may result in torsades de pointes or other arrhythmias.
12) **Correct answer: C |** The proper initial treatment is based on stabilization of the extremity by immobilizing the affected leg below the level of the heart. This can help minimize the distribution of venom. Poison control does not recommend applying ice to the affected area as some believe.
13) **Correct answer: A |** Bath salts closely exhibit amphetamines. These drugs are synthetic cathinones, the active ingredient in the Khat plant. The Khat plant is chewed in the Middle East for their stimulant effects. This plant mimics amphetamines and cocaine by causing rapid alterations in the serum levels of dopamine and serotonin.
14) **Correct answer: D |** In a pediatric patient that's positive for herpes, the proper first action is standard room isolation and normal universal precautions.

Chapter 12 | Neonatal Defects & Surgical Emergencies

1) **Correct answer: D |** Intussusception is a condition that causes telescoping of the bowels. This can commonly cause secondary ischemia and death. The infant will present with nausea, vomiting and "jelly stools". Exam will reveal a palpable sausage mass on abdominal exam. Correction is completed by barium enema, manual manipulation or full bowel resection.

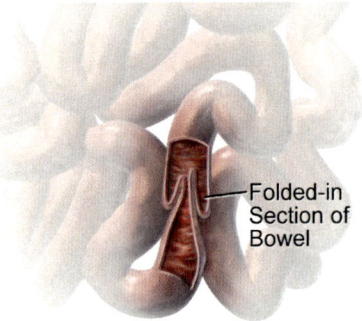

Intussusception of the Bowel

Bruce Blaus Blausen.com staff (2014). "Medical gallery of Blausen Medical 2014". WikiJournal of Medicine 1 (2)

2) **Correct answer: A |** This is classic for pyloric stenosis. Pyloric stenosis is where the pyloric sphincter is pathologically narrow and hinders the stomach contents from passing into the intestines. Treatment will consist of surgical intervention, supportive care, fluid hydration and electrolyte evaluation/correction.

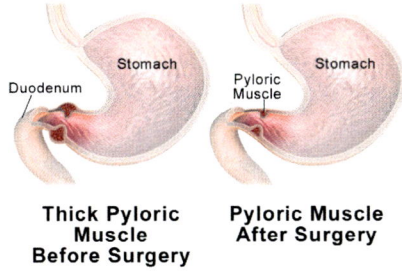

Thick Pyloric Muscle Before Surgery   Pyloric Muscle After Surgery

Bruce Blaus Blausen.com staff (2014). "Medical gallery of Blausen Medical 2014". WikiJournal of Medicine 1 (2)

3) **Correct answer: C |** This presents as a hole between the trachea and esophagus. The neonate will present with large amounts of oral secretions, coughing, and choking. Treatment is supportive until surgical intervention can be completed. No feeding. Intubation with secondary NG/OG tube placement is key.

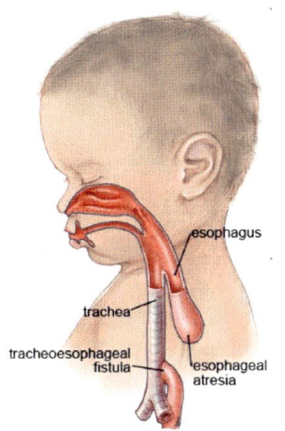

Most common form (90% to 95%) of tracheoesophageal fistula. Upper segment of esophagus ending in blind pouch; lower segment originating from trachea just above bifurcation. The two segments may be connected by a solid cord

https://tefnormalanatomy.wordpress.com/2012/04/29/tracheoesophageal-fistula/

4) **Correct answer: D |** Choanal atresia is a narrowing or blockage of tissue in the nasal airways. These patients will have difficulty breathing and inability to nurse and breath at the same time. Diagnosis is made by attempting to pass a small suction catheter through the nares. Surgical intervention is indicated to repair and remove the blockage in the back of the nasal passages.

5) **Correct answer: B** | Transposition of the great vessels is a severe diagnosis for any neonate. It's often associated with a VSD and/or PDA patency. It's essential for the PDA to remain patent for the survival of the baby. Often times they will surgically cause a VSD just to provide some oxygen rich blood to flow through the body. These patients are hypoxic and very sick.
6) **Correct answer: C** | This is a quick calculation for determining tube size on the fly for pediatrics > 1 year. You can also use the Broselow tape or the baby's pinky finger.
7) **Correct answer: B** | Prostaglandin can cause significant respiratory depression and apnea in neonates. This is most often dose dependent. This doesn't mean you intubate automatically, just be ready and prepared. Remember to always calculate your O_2 because too much oxygen will cause PDA closure. With these neonates, survival is dependent on PDA patency until surgical intervention is completed.
   Calculation equation:
   $$\frac{\%FiO_2 \times P1}{P2} = FiO_2 \text{ at new altitude}$$
   - P1 = Current barometric pressure
   - P2 = New barometric pressure at altitude
8) **Correct answer: C** | Neonates and pediatrics compensate well. Remember that you will only see decompensation after 25% blood loss. In a neonate that may only be 10-20mLs. Normal circulating blood supply is 75-80 mL/kg.
9) **Correct answer: D** | Subtle seizures consist of repetitive mouth/tongue movements, bicycling, eye deviation and blinking. Clonic seizures include repetitive jerky movements of limbs. Tonic seizures may resemble posturing or tonic extension seen in older patients. Myoclonic seizures include multiple jerking motions, usually of the upper extremities.
10) **Correct answer: C** | Pulmonary arterial vasoconstriction keeps blood from flowing through the fetal lungs and causes oxygenation to take place in the placenta. At birth, pulmonary adaptation occurs after a complex series of events switches respiration from the placenta to the lungs.

11) **Correct answer: C** | Stress on a neonate can present in many different ways. One of those would be the baby suddenly starts hiccoughing, yawning or sneezing multiple times. Although these things can be found normally in the neonate, with distress these things will occur multiple times in a row and all of a sudden.
12) **Correct answer: A** | Subtle seizure activity can present in many forms in the neonate and infant. Increasing HR and BP as well as eye fluttering, mouth movements and bicycling actions are also signs of seizure activity within the neonate. You may also see an increase in irritability and decrease in SpO_2 during seizure activity.
13) **Correct answer: B** | Surfactant is absent in very premature babies and is required to keep the lungs inflated and keep them from sticking. Surfactant helps keep the alveoli open. Without sufficient surfactant, alveolar collapse, atelectasis trauma and respiratory distress will ensue.
14) **Correct answer: C** | In some cases, a patent PDA is beneficial to the neonate and may prolong their life until surgical correction is possible. Prostaglandin administration allows the ductus arteriosus to remain open. Indomethacin blocks prostaglandin production and is used for closure of PDA.
15) **Correct answer: C** | Patients that suffer from Tetralogy of Fallot have multiple issues. Most often, they suffer from a VSD, stenotic pulmonary valve, RV hypertrophy and a pulmonary artery outflow obstruction. PDA patency is essential. Administration of oxygen needs to be minimal along with prostaglandin (PGE1) administration throughout transport. A potential side effect to PGE1 administration is apnea. Intubation is not essential but the clinician should be alert and ready for any complications that may arise. Long-term treatment is dilation of the pulmonary artery to alleviate the PA outflow obstruction and surgical repair of the VSD.
16) **Correct answer: C** | Tetralogy of Fallot is a right-to-left shunt allowing blood to flow from the right heart to the left heart. Tetralogy of Fallot results in four defects including: pulmonary stenosis, overriding aorta, right ventricular hypertrophy and ventricular septal defect.

17) **Correct answer: B** | Prior to birth, the placenta is a major source of prostaglandin to keep the PDA open. At birth, pulmonary vascular resistance decreases and blood flows directly from the right ventricle into the lungs. Normal respiration and oxygen tension increases as well causing closure of the PDA.

18) **Correct answer: D** | VSD is one of the most common congenital heart defects, and occurs when there is a hole in the septum between the left and right ventricles.

19) **Correct answer: C** | Proper ETT sizing for pediatric patients should be calculated using: (Age + 16) / 4.

20) **Correct answer: C** | Depth of insertion of an ETT should be approximately 3x that of the ETT size.

21) **Correct answer: D** | Forceful bilious vomiting is the hallmark of a volvulus and should immediately increase your index of suspicion toward this diagnosis. X-ray will show a dilated stomach, with large amounts of air in the small intestine. With a volvulus, there's a very high risk of sepsis. As such, NG/OG tube placement, fluids and broad-spectrum antibiotics should be started.

22) **Correct answer: C** | Necrotizing enterocolitis is the most common neonatal GI medical/surgical emergency. These patients present with abdominal distension and curvilinear pneumatosis intestinalis (presence of gas within the small and large intestine). Labs will show leukopenia, thrombocytopenia and metabolic acidosis. This disease is highly fatal, with a mortality rate >50%.

23) **Correct answer: D** | Hirschsprung's disease presents in the neonate when they are unable to pass meconium in the first two days of life. The neonate will present with abdominal swelling and possible vomiting. X-ray will show gaseous dilated bowel. The disease manifests from nerve cells that do not develop normally along the bowel resulting in the failure of the colon to relax and the inability to pass stool. Fluid resuscitation, malabsorption, and malnutrition should be aggressively assessed until medical management or possible surgical repair can be completed.

Hirschsprung Example

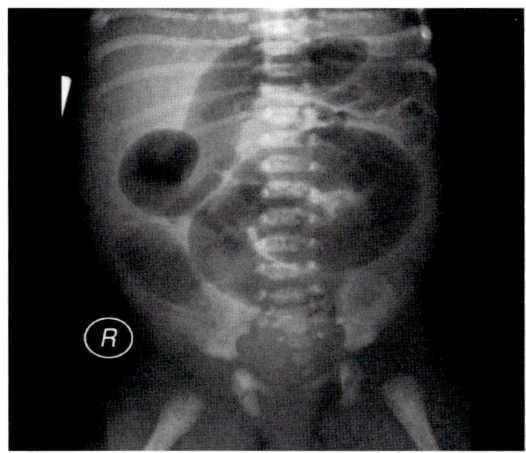

https://radiopaedia.org/cases/hirschsprung-disease-1

24) **Correct answer: D |** Omphalocele is a defect in the abdominal wall that can result in bowel ischemia and/or death. Assessment reveals a protruding, encapsulated intestine. This is however often found during prenatal screening and the doctor and parents are normally aware of the defect prior to birth. Repair can be difficult due to lack of development of the abdominal cavity. Heat loss is a major concern, and a radiant warmer, warm fluids and wrapped torso are essential initial treatments.

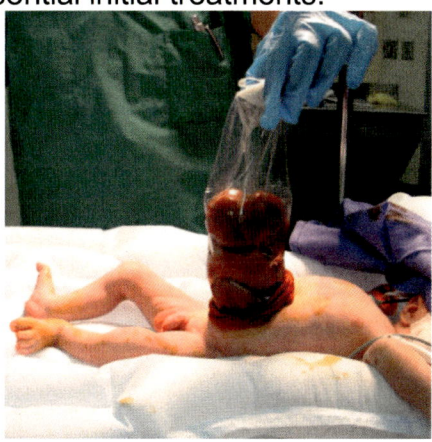

https://online.epocrates.com/diseases/115871/Omphalocele-and-gastroschisis/Image-Library

25) **Correct Answer: D |** The best position for a neonate with a myelomeningocele is to place them prone with knees abducted, thus taking pressure off the myelomeningocele. This also allows for optimal positioning of the hips, knees and feet because orthopedic problems are common.

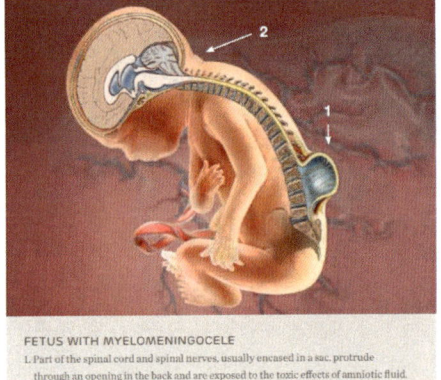

TYPES OF SPINA BIFIDA
- Myelomeningocele (MMC) ▶
- Myeloschisis
- Lipomeningocele
- Myelocystocele

Open neural tube defects such as myelomeningocele and myeloschisis are treatable by fetal repair.

Closed neural tube defects such as lipomeningocele and myelocystocele are not treatable by fetal repair.

FETUS WITH MYELOMENINGOCELE
1. Part of the spinal cord and spinal nerves, usually encased in a sac, protrude through an opening in the back and are exposed to the toxic effects of amniotic fluid.
2. Arnold-Chiari II Malformation: Cerebrospinal fluid (CSF) leaks through the opening in the back, and the brain stem (hindbrain) descends, or herniates, into the spinal canal in the neck and blocks the circulation of CSF. This can cause a damaging buildup of fluid in the brain called hydrocephalus.

https://issuu.com/choppublications/docs/spina-bifida-flip-book/3

Chapter 15 | Study Tips

1. The C-NPT exam is multiple choice and only has A, B, & C choices.
2. Study and sufficiently prepare.
3. Take notes during your study sessions and go back and review those notes.
4. Go back and find weak areas and focus on them.
5. Time management – be sure to know how much time can be spent on each question.
6. If you have the ability to go back, write down questions you were unsure about and go back and look at them again instead of staying on the question too long. Limit (1) minute per question.
7. Most of the time, these tests allow you more than enough time to finish the exam.
8. Be sure to read the question slowly and fully to understand what is being asked of you.
9. Beware of distractors – don't get caught up in the scenario. Read the last couple of sentences to determine what is being asked of you.
10. Pay close attention to phrases such as: EXCEPT.
11. <u>Eliminate the distractors and wrong answers first; this usually leaves you with two good answers. Be able to select the best answer of the two.</u>
12. Think about your answer before you look at the choices; this may help you with the correct answer or to jog your memory to determine the correct answer.
13. There are usually trigger words in questions to make you automatically think of the answer. C/P that is stabbing and radiating into the back – think aneurysm. Referred (L) shoulder pain – think spleen.
14. Use the paper or board supplied to you for quick numbers you want to remember.
15. Hit problem areas right before the test and write down any numbers or values that you think might help you.
16. Get plenty of rest and eat a good breakfast

FlightBridgeED, LLC
References

Alspach, J. (Ed.). (1998). *Core curriculum for critical care nursing* (6th Ed.). Philadelphia, PA: Saunders Elsevier

American College of Surgeons (2012). *Advanced trauma life support student course manual* 9th Ed. Philadelphia: Lippincott, Williams & Wilkins

American Heart Association & American Academy of Pediatrics. (2000). *Neonatal resuscitation textbook* (4th Ed.). Elk Grove Village: American Academy of Pediatrics

ARDS Network. (1998). *Prospective, randomized, multi-center trial of 12 ml/kg vs. 6 ml/kg tidal volume positive pressure ventilation for treatment of acute lung injury and acute respiratory distress syndrome (ARMA).* ARDSNet Study 01, Version III. Retrieved from http://www.ardsnet.org/system/files/armaprotocolV3_1998-09-11_0.pdf

Darovic, G. (2002). *Hemodynamic monitoring invasive and non-invasive clinical application* 3rd Ed. Philadelphia: W.B. Saunders Co

Dellinger, R., Mitchell, L. M., Rhodes, A., Annane, D., Gerlach, H., & Opal, S. M. (2013, February). Surviving sepsis campaign: international guidelines for management of severe sepsis and septic shock: 2012. *Critical Care Medicine, 41*(2), 580-636. Retrieved from www.ccmjournal.org

Guy, J. (2007, March 13). Oxygenation and PEEP. ICU Rounds Podcast. Nashville, TN, USA.

Fischbach, F. (2004). *A manual of laboratory and diagnostic tests* (7th Ed.). Philadelphia, PA: Lippincott Williams & Wilkins

Guyton, A., & Hall, J. (2000). *Textbook of medical physiology* (10th Ed.). Philadelphia, PA: W.B. Saunders Elsevier

Holleran, R. (Ed.). (2005). *Air and surface patient transport: Principles & practice* (3rd Ed.). Philadelphia, PA: Elsevier Health Sciences

Holleran, R. (Ed.). (2010). *Air and surface patient transport: Principles & practice* (4th Ed.). Philadelphia, PA: Elsevier Health Sciences

Kattwinkel J. (Ed.) (2006). Neonatal resuscitation textbook 5th Ed. Dallas: American Academy of Pediatrics & American Heart Association

Marino, P. L. (1998). *The ICU book* (2nd ed.). (S. R. Zinner, Ed.) Baltimore, MD: Lippincott Williams & Wilkins

McIntosh, L. (1997). *Essentials of nurse anesthesia.* New York: McGraw-Hill Companies Inc.

Mejia, R. (Ed.). (2008). *Pediatric fundamental critical care support.* Mount Prospect, IL: Society of Critcal Care Medicine

Neligan, P. (2006). Acute Lung Injury. Retrieved from Critical Care Medicine Tutorials: http://www.ccmtutorials.com/rs/ali/vili.htm

Neligan, P. (2006, December). Critical Care Medicine Tutorials. Retrieved from All about Oxygen: http://www.ccmtutorials.com/index.htm

Nolan, P.J. (Ed.). (1995). *Fundamentals of college physics*. Dubuque, IA: Wm. C. Brown Communications, Inc.

Madden Maureen A. (2013) *Pediatric Fundamentals Of Critical Care Support* (2nd Ed), Society of Critical Care Medicine

Pillitteri A. (2007). *Maternal & child health nursing* (5th Ed.). Philadelphia, PA: Lippincott, Williams & Wilkins

Pollack, Andrew. (Ed.). (2010). *Critical Care Transport*. Sudbury, MA: Jones and Bartlett Publishers

Karlson, Kristen (2012) *S.T.A.B.L.E*, American Academy of Pediatrics

Surgeons, A. A. (2011). Critical Care Transport. In A. Pollack. Jones and Bartlett Learning. Retrieved from: http://www.aic.cuhk.edu.hk/web8/prvc.htm

Tintinalli, J., Kelen, G. Stapczynski, J. (Ed.). (2004) Emergency medicine: A comprehensive study guide 6th Ed. New York: McGraw-Hill Companies Inc.

Urden, L., Stacy, K., & Lough, M. (2005). *Thelan's critical care nursing diagnosis and management* (5th Ed.). Maryland Heights, MO: Elsevier Health Sciences

Walls, R., Murphy, M., Luten, R., & Schneider, R. (2008). *The manual of emergency airway management.* (3rd Ed.). Philadelphia, PA: Lippincott Williams & Wilkin

Picture References

https://www.researchgate.net/figure/Acute-respiratory-distress-syndrome-with-widespread-ground-glass-opacity-and-air_fig1_50249686

http://www.adhb.govt.nz/newborn/TeachingResources/Radiology/CXR/OtherCHF/NonstructuralCHF.jpg

https://radiopaedia.org/cases/congenital-diaphragmatic-hernia

https://en.wikipedia.org/wiki/Steeple_sign

http://learningradiology.com/archives04/COW%20108-Epiglottitis/epiglottitiscorrect.htm

https://radiopaedia.org/articles/tension-pneumothorax

Bruce Blaus Blausen.com staff (2014). "Medical gallery of Blausen Medical 2014". WikiJournal of Medicine 1 (2)

https://tefnormalanatomy.wordpress.com/2012/04/29/tracheoesophageal-fistula/

https://online.epocrates.com/diseases/115871/Omphalocele-and-gastroschisis/Image-Library

https://issuu.com/choppublications/docs/spina-bifida-flip-book/3

Made in the USA
Monee, IL
03 October 2025